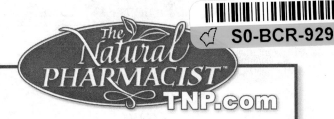

The Natural PHARMACIST™
TNP.com

Inside—Find the Answers to These Questions and More

☑ Can echinacea reduce my cold and flu symptoms? (See page 20.)

☑ Will it help me get over a cold or flu faster? (See page 17.)

☑ What's the proper dose of echinacea? (See page 28.)

☑ Which type of echinacea should I use? (See page 18.)

☑ Are there any side effects? (See page 28.)

☑ Why is echinacea not the best choice for preventing colds? (See page 23.)

☑ Can ginseng help prevent colds? (See page 75.)

☑ Can vitamin E improve immunity? (See page 93.)

☑ Can andrographis reduce cold symptoms? (See page 52.)

☑ What form of zinc should be used for colds? (See page 41.)

THE NATURAL PHARMACIST™ Library

Feverfew and Migraines

Heart Disease Prevention

Kava and Anxiety

Natural Health Bible

Natural Treatments for Arthritis

Natural Treatments for Colds and Flus

Natural Treatments for Diabetes

Natural Treatments for High Cholesterol

Natural Treatments to Improve Memory

Natural Treatments for Menopause

PMS

Reducing Cancer Risk

Saw Palmetto and the Prostate

St. John's Wort and Depression

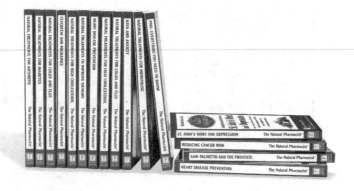

To order, visit www.TNP.com

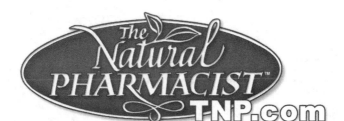

Natural Treatments for Colds and Flus

Anna M. Barton
Elizabeth Collins, N.D.
Nancy Berkoff, R.D., Ed.D.

Series Editors

Steven Bratman, M.D.
David Kroll, Ph.D.

A DIVISION OF PRIMA PUBLISHING
3000 Lava Ridge Court ■ Roseville, California 95661
(800) 632-8676 ■ www.TNP.com

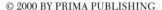

© 2000 BY PRIMA PUBLISHING

Published in association with TNP.com.

Warning—Disclaimer

TNP.COM, THENATURALPHARMACIST.COM, THE NATURAL PHARMACIST, and PRIMA HEALTH are trademarks of Prima Communications Inc. The Prima colophon is a trademark of Prima Communications Inc., registered with the United States Patent and Trademark Office.

The Food and Drug Administration has not approved the use of any of the natural treatments discussed in this book. This book, and the information contained herein, has not been approved by the Food and Drug Administration.

Pseudonyms have been used throughout to protect the privacy of the individuals involved.

All products mentioned in this book are trademarks of their respective companies.

Illustrations by Helene Stevens. Illustrations © 1999 by Prima Publishing. All rights reserved.

Library of Congress Cataloging-in-Publication Data
Barton, Anna M.
    The natural pharmacist : natural treatments for colds and flus / Anna M. Barton, Elizabeth Collins, Nancy Berkoff.
        p.   cm. — (The natural pharmacist)
    Includes bibliographical references and index.
    ISBN 0-7615-2469-X
        1. Influenza—Alternative treatment. 2. Cold (Disease)—Alternative treatment. I. Title.
    II. Series.
RC150 . B33   1999
616.2'0506--dc21   99-057540
               00 01 02 HH 10 9 8 7 6 5 4 3 2 1
               Printed in the United States of America

How to Order
Single copies may be ordered from Prima Publishing, 3000 Lava Ridge Court, Roseville, CA 95661; telephone (800) 632-8676. Quantity discounts are also available. On your letterhead, include information concerning the intended use of the books and the number of books you wish to purchase.

Visit us online at www.TNP.com and www.primahealth.com

Contents

What Makes This Book Different?

The interest in natural medicine has never been greater. According to the National Association of Chain Drug Stores, 65 million Americans are using natural supplements, and the number is growing! Yet, it is hard for the consumer to find trustworthy sources for balanced information about this emerging field. Why? Frankly, natural medicine has had a checkered history. From snake oil potions sold at the turn of the century to those books, magazines, and product catalogs that hype miracle cures today, this is a field where exaggerated claims have been the norm. Proponents of natural medicine have tended to abuse science, treating it more as a marketing tool than a means of discovering the truth.

But there is truth to be found. Studies of vitamins, minerals, and other food supplements have been with us since these nutritional substances were first discovered, and the level and quality of this science has grown dramatically in the last 20 years. Herbal medicine has been neglected in the United States, but in Europe, this, the oldest of all healing arts, has been the subject of tremendous and ongoing scientific interest.

At present, for a number of herbs and supplements, it is possible to give reasonably scientific answers to the questions: How well does this work? How safe is it? What types of conditions is it best used for?

THE NATURAL PHARMACIST series is designed to cut through the hype and tell you what is known and what remains to be scientifically proven regarding popular natural treatments. These books are more conservative than any others available, more honest about the weaknesses of natural approaches, more fair in their comparisons of natural and conventional treatments. You won't find any miracle cures here, but you will discover useful options that can help you become healthier.

Why Choose Natural Treatments?

Although the science behind natural medicine continues to grow, this is still a much less scientifically validated field than conventional medicine. You might ask, "Why should I resort to an herb that is only partly proven, when I could take a drug with solid science behind it?" There are at least three good reasons to consider natural alternatives.

First, some herbs and supplements offer benefits that are not matched by any conventional drug. Vitamin E is a good example. It appears to help prevent prostate cancer, a benefit that no standard medication can claim. Also, vitamin E almost certainly helps prevent heart disease. While there are standard drugs that also prevent heart disease, vitamin E works differently and may be able to complement many of the other approaches.

Another example is the herb milk thistle. Studies strongly suggest that this herb can protect the liver from injury. There is no pill or tablet your doctor can prescribe to do the same.

Even if the science behind some of these treatments is less than perfect, when the risks are low and the possible benefit high, a natural treatment may be worth trying. It is a little-known fact that for many conventional treatments the science is less than perfect as well, and physicians must balance uncertain benefits against incompletely understood risks.

A second reason to consider natural therapies is that some may offer benefits comparable to those of drugs with fewer side effects. The herb St. John's wort is a good example. Reasonably strong scientific evidence suggests that this herb is an effective treatment for mild to moderate depression, while producing fewer side effects on average than conventional medications. Saw palmetto for benign enlargement of the prostate, ginkgo for relieving symptoms and perhaps slowing the progression of Alzheimer's disease, and glucosamine for osteoarthritis are other examples. This is not to say that herbs and supplements are completely harmless—they're not—but for most the level of risk is quite low.

Finally, there is a philosophical point to consider. For many people, it "feels" better to use a treatment that comes from nature instead of from a laboratory. Just as you might rather wear all-cotton clothing than polyester, or look at a mountain landscape rather than the skyscrapers of a downtown city, natural treatments may simply feel more compatible with your view of life. We can quibble endlessly about just what "natural" means and whether a certain treatment is "actually" natural or not, but such arguments are beside the point. The difference is in the feeling, and feelings matter. In fact, having a good feeling about taking an herb may lead you to use it more consistently than you would a prescription drug.

Of course, at times synthetic drugs may be necessary and even lifesaving. But on many other occasions it may be quite reasonable to turn to an herb or supplement instead of a drug.

To make good decisions you need good information. Unfortunately, while hundreds of books on alternative medicine are published every year, many are highly misleading. The phrase "studies prove" is often used when the studies in question are so small or so badly conducted that they prove nothing at all. You may even find that the "data" from other books comes from studies with petri dishes and not real people!

You can't even assume that books written by well-known authors are scientifically sound. Many of these authors rely on secondary writers, leading to a game of "telephone," where misconceptions are passed around from book to book. And there's a strong tendency to exaggerate the power of natural remedies, whitewashing them with selective reporting.

THE NATURAL PHARMACIST series gives you the balanced information you need to make informed decisions about your health needs. Setting a new, high standard of accuracy and objectivity, these books take a realistic look at the herbs and supplements you read about in the news. You will encounter both favorable and unfavorable studies in these pages and will learn about both the benefits and the risks of natural treatments.

THE NATURAL PHARMACIST series is the source you can trust.

Steven Bratman, M.D.
David Kroll, Ph.D.

Introduction

N ow and then you run across one of those people who likes to announce—as you bury your miserable, red, stuffy nose into your tissue for the fifty-thousandth time—that they *never* get colds. But such people are rare (possibly because they take their lives in their hands making such statements to those who are suffering). At the opposite end of the spectrum are people who just can't seem to stay healthy for more than a few weeks at a time, especially through the winter months. If you're not among the rare birds who simply stay healthy all the time, this book probably contains some information that can help you. We can't promise that you'll become one of those disgustingly healthy people who never get sick, but you can likely reduce the frequency and severity of the illnesses you do experience.

As you no doubt already know, the over-the-counter drugs available for cold treatment won't shorten your cold any; all they can do is treat the symptoms. Often the drowsiness these medications cause is as much a deterrent to getting your work done as the cold symptoms themselves. For flus there is a bit more hope offered by conventional medicine in the form of vaccines and drugs that will help to prevent you from getting sick, or reduce your symptoms and recovery time if you do—at least for certain types of flus.

Other options for treating or preventing colds and flus are herbs and supplements that appear to boost your body's own defenses in fighting off diseases. For instance, there is evidence that certain herbs and supplements such as echinacea, andrographis, zinc, and vitamin C may actually reduce the length of time you are sick, as well as the severity of your symptoms. So suppose you do start coming down with the flu—but you immediately start taking echinacea. Research suggests that instead of feeling really rotten for the next eight days, you may not feel quite so bad, and you could start to recover in only four days. You still may have a bit of stuffy nose and sore throat. But it could mean that you feel well enough to keep working on that presentation you're supposed to give at the end of the week and can actually be there to present it. This is a lot better than having to make excuses to your boss—and then having to deal with the stress *that* brings on while you're trying to recuperate.

Within the pages of this book are answers to questions like "What is the difference between a cold and the flu?" "What is 'Indian echinacea,' and can it really help prevent colds?" "Do zinc lozenges help treat sore throats or not?" We'll give you understandable, unbiased reporting of the scientific research on using herbs and supplements for colds and flus: Which ones relieve symptoms and help you get well quicker? Which may actually prevent you from getting sick to begin with? Which just don't seem to work? We'll also provide information on the proper dosage and safety for these natural alternatives to conventional medicine. Our goal is to equip you with the knowledge you need to make educated choices about caring for yourself and your family during the cold and flu season. Welcome!

CHAPTER
ONE

About Colds
and Flus

I t's a good bet that you already know something about colds and flus—you've probably had your share. However, many people are confused about the difference between a cold and the flu, while some use the terms interchangeably. There are some differences, though, and in some cases how you decide to treat your illness will depend on which you have. Therefore, let's start with the basics: Know your enemy.

We know that the common cold is caused by many different viruses. There are more than 100 varieties of "rhinoviruses" (the largest group of cold-causing viruses). Medical books describe the common cold as an acute, self-limiting infection of the upper respiratory tract: sore throat, sneezing, headache, congestion, runny nose, and fatigue—all of which will go away in due time.

I Opened the Window, and Influenza

Remember the old punch line to the joke where a student is asked to use the word "influenza" in a sentence? Many of the treatments that work for colds work for flus as well. As you may already know, "flu" is short for "influenza," a more serious type of disease than the common cold. The flu is caused by a different group of viruses than are colds. Influenza occurs in three main classifications: type A, type B, and type C. Of the three, type A is by far the most common, as well as the most potentially severe; type B is the second most common; and type C is relatively uncommon. The influenza A virus spontaneously changes a little from year to year, which is why you need a new vaccination every year. When it changes a great deal during a particular year, there is a more severe epidemic because people's natural resistance developed from last year's flu doesn't protect them. Occasionally, major changes occur, at which time we experience worldwide super-epidemics called pandemics that can kill millions of people.

The symptoms of influenza are similar to those of the common cold but almost always more severe.

Most years, the flu arrives in the late fall or early winter. The symptoms of influenza are similar to those of the common cold but almost always more severe. The onset is usually sudden, with fever up to 103°F (39°C), severe exhaustion, and muscle and joint aches (especially in the back and legs) in addition to a prominent headache, runny nose, sore throat, and possibly a cough. As the illness progresses, the muscle aches tend to get worse, and the cough becomes more prominent. You may notice that you're sensitive to light, your eyes may water, and you may even experience nausea and vomiting. While the majority of these symptoms should abate in a few days to a week, you may find that your fatigue and weakness linger and that you tend to sweat easily for weeks.

Influenza can be dangerous for the very young and very old, women in the third trimester of pregnancy, and those with lung disease, heart disease, kidney disease, diabetes, blood diseases (such as sickle-cell anemia), or immunosuppression (as with AIDS or leukemia). Herbs and supplements are not adequate treatment for people in these high-risk groups.

Flus can worsen chronic respiratory illnesses (like asthma and bronchitis), possibly leading to hospitalization. Sometimes, flus can cause their own form of pneumonia, which usually requires hospitalization. Rare complications of flus include (but are not limited to) encephalitis (inflammation of the brain), myocarditis and pericarditis (inflammations of the heart), and Guillain-Barré syndrome. It is not clear whether any natural treatments can reduce the risk of these complications.

Neither Colds Nor Flus

Sometimes, it isn't clear whether what you have is a cold or a flu. A bad cold might feel a lot like a mild flu and vice versa. In addition, numerous other viruses produce symptoms that don't fit exactly into either camp. Bacterial infections can also produce similar, although in many ways more intense, symptoms. Such diseases as a sinus infection, bronchitis, pneumonia, or strep throat are often caused not by viruses but by bacteria.

Back in the old days, before antibiotics had been discovered, some herbal remedies were used to treat bacterial infections. However, it's important to remember that in those times it was not uncommon for people to die when they got pneumonia or some such bacterial illness.

In any case, with antibiotics being so effective and easily available, trying herbal alternatives is not advisable unless the bacterial infection is fairly mild.

Bacterial infections can produce symptoms similar to, although in many ways more intense than, viral infections.

The treatments discussed in this book are aimed at treating the types of viruses that cause flus and colds. These treatments could in some cases provide some symptomatic relief or a little boost to your immune system that might help your body overcome a mild bacterial infection without having to resort to antibiotics.

But before we go on to talk about the treatments available, let's learn a little about the ways the "villains," viruses and bacteria, work to invade our bodies. It will help us understand why the two really need different treatments.

Viruses

Viruses are very bizarre organisms. Actually it's not even certain whether viruses can be considered organisms because they lack several of the characteristics generally thought essential for something to be considered "alive." For instance, they cannot have offspring in the normal sense. They don't have any metabolic function of their own—meaning they don't eat, breathe, or grow. But, like little robots, they invade the machinery in our cells and slip a set of instructions for making more, identical little robots into our DNA, and then our own cells obligingly build armies of them!

How do they do it? Well, our cells are very much like little factories. Cells making up the different parts of our bodies specialize in making proteins that we need for each location. For instance, some of the cells in our eyes produce the secretions we need to keep our eyes moist, while certain cells in the pancreas make enzymes that digest our foods. Each cell knows what to make by "reading" the appropriate sections of our DNA, a form of a chemical—nucleic acid—that acts as the software that contains the programming for our bodies.

Virus particles consist only of a protein coating containing nucleic acid—either DNA or RNA. If "read" by the machinery in your cell, this viral nucleic acid is translated into a set of instructions for building more viruses. Viruses sneak past the cell membrane, and once inside the cell, they shed their coats. This lets the nucleic acid out of the protein coat. It's like slipping the wrong software into a computer—which is why computer viruses were named after them.

Your unsuspecting cell will build so many of these viruses that it fills, like a balloon, until it pops, spilling millions of viruses out into your bloodstream. These viruses then seek out and infiltrate new cells.

The Body's Defense

Have you ever seen one of those movies where they have a hostage situation in some nice building and the S.W.A.T. team comes to the rescue? They save the hostages, they get rid of the bad guys—but wouldn't you hate to be the landlord! Sometimes our own immune systems also cause a lot of damage while trying to help.

Our immune systems see these viral invaders and charge in to do something about them. Our S.W.A.T. team raises our body temperature to destroy them, sends special cells that will engulf and consume them (which can also cause inflammation), and produces mucus secretions to try to wash them out. If you were a member of an invading army and you saw a wave of mucus oozing up out of the floor, engulfing your fellow soldiers and sweeping them toward the exit, wouldn't you find that formidable? It's really our bodies' attempts to rid us of the virus that we perceive as symptoms.

Secondary Infections: Adding Insult to Injury

Some viruses can leave us more susceptible to invasion by bacteria as well. For instance, damage to the cells lining your nose, throat, or lungs might make it easier for a *Streptococcus* bacteria to take up housekeeping. It's sort of like leaving the door standing open. This is yet another good reason to try to minimize the amount of time you keep that virus around. The

Zinc lozenges may be one way to help you avoid a bacterial infection.

sooner it's gone, the sooner you can "lock up." Zinc lozenges, which we'll talk about in chapter 4, may be one way to evict your unwanted viral "tenants," and this could help you avoid a bacterial infection.

Bacteria

Bacteria, unlike viruses, are definitely leading little lives of their own. They make all their own proteins; they eat, grow, breed, and so forth. Fortunately for us, there are some major differences between bacteria and humans. Besides the obvious ones, such as *our* ability to enjoy shopping, chocolate, football, or philosophy, some bacteria produce enzymes we can't produce, even though we need them to help us digest our foods. These sorts of bacteria normally live inside us and are essential to our survival. Another reason to celebrate our differences, though, is that bacteria have some important structural differences from our cells that allow us to kill them with antibiotics without killing ourselves. This is useful when one of the nasty types invades our systems.

The nasty types—pathogenic bacteria—seem to think of us the way Columbus and his cohorts thought of the American continents. Notwithstanding the fact that we are already inhabited, they are ready and willing to move in and help themselves to our resources.

The suggestions in this book for improving your resistance to illnesses may help you avoid getting sick so often, whether the cause is a virus or a form of bacteria. If you have a serious bacterial infection, however, antibiotics can be lifesaving (see chapter 10 for more information).

Reducing Cold and Flu Symptoms

In the following chapters, we cover the herbs and supplements that have been found to reduce the discomfort and length of viral upper respiratory infections (like echinacea and andrographis, among others), as well as some that may help in preventing illness (like ginseng). In chapter 9, we cover some of the basic, commonsense sorts of things you can do to avoid getting sick in the first place or to relieve your symptoms until you're well.

The main use for the herbs and supplements we'll discuss in these chapters is for treating viruses that cause the symptoms we refer to as flus and colds. But remember: Limiting viral infections may also help you sidestep a secondary infection caused by bacteria, and that's worth doing.

We're used to going down the aisles at the local pharmacy and seeing a huge section of treatments for cold and flu symptoms—multiple over-the-counter remedies, and several brands of each one. You can buy capsules to loosen your phlegm, syrup to stop your cough, pills for itchy nose and watery eyes, sprays for clogged-up noses . . . the list goes on and on.

These over-the-counter medications may slightly reduce cold and flu symptoms once you have the illness, but that's about all they do. They won't kill the virus that's infecting you or help you get over the cold any faster. And no medication will prevent your catching a cold in the first place.

If you specifically have influenza A or B, the situation is a little better. Certain prescription medications *can* help you get better faster, if you take them within a few days of your first symptoms. Two of these medications can also help prevent influenza A, and the newest of the group, like the flu vaccine, can ward off both influenza A and B. But once a cold or flu is well established, the best advice your doctor will offer is that you should rest, drink lots of fluids, take acetaminophen for the headache, and wait for it to end.

Wouldn't it be nice if, as you shuffle down the aisle with your nose buried in your handkerchief, you could find something to help you recover faster? Well you can. But instead of heading for an over-the-counter or prescription drug, you're more likely to find relief by trying one of the natural herbs or supplements described in this book.

Zinc seems to help you get better faster if you treat the cold right at the start.

Good evidence suggests that echinacea, andrographis, and vitamin C can all help you recover faster. In addition, the mineral zinc seems to be able to do for colds what those prescription medications do for influenza A—help you get better faster if you treat the cold right at the start. And other treatments may be able to help prevent both colds and flus, something no drug or vaccine can do as yet. We'll start with the herbs, vitamins, and minerals for which the research evidence is strongest. Then we'll work our way down to those that have some reputation but that may not have been seriously studied well enough for us to know how effective they actually are. In this chapter, we give a brief overview of the options that exist. The following chapters will focus in more detail on the remedies.

Echinacea: A Great American Tradition

If echinacea were the bragging type, it could mention that its ancestors were here before anyone arrived on the *Mayflower*—and so could the people who originally used this herb for medicinal purposes. Echinacea is a flowering plant native to North America, a relative of asters and daisies. Native Americans, and later European settlers and their descendants, have used it for a wide variety of illnesses and injuries, including snakebites, which is how it came by one of its nicknames: snakeroot.

At least nine double-blind placebo-controlled studies (for definition of these terms, see "Scientific Method," page 13) have been done on the effects of orally ingested (taken by mouth) echinacea on cold and flu symptoms. Most of these have found that echinacea shortened the duration and/or reduced the severity of symptoms. (Regular use of echinacea, however, does not seem to *prevent* colds, as you'll see below.)

For more detail about the plant, its history, the research that has been done on it, and how to use it, see chapter 2.

Vitamin C: It Isn't Just for Breakfast Anymore

A great deal of research has focused on the functions of vitamin C. Part of what we've learned is that it does appear to help

Taking It on Faith

Despite the fact that the research done on echinacea and vitamin C suggests that neither is effective (except in certain situations) in preventing colds and flus, some people still use them for that purpose. One man who takes both echinacea and vitamin C swears they are the reason he hasn't had a cold in years.

On the surface, he may seem to be living proof that the studies are wrong. After all, not having a single cold in a number of years *is* unusual! But from a researcher's point of view, this doesn't prove that echinacea and vitamin C are responsible. For one thing, we can't know for sure whether he would have gotten any colds had he not been taking these substances. Perhaps he just has a very healthy immune system.

Or it's possible that he is demonstrating the most positive aspects of the placebo effect (see "The Power of Suggestion: Placebos and Double-Blinding," page 13). Because he truly believes he will not get a cold or flu while taking echinacea and vitamin C, he subconsciously activates his own immune system.

make colds shorter and less severe; it may also help "abort" a cold that is just starting. As everyone knows, vitamin C is found in citrus fruit, but it is also an ingredient in broccoli, red peppers, strawberries, brussels sprouts, parsley, and currants. And, of course, it's available in supplement form.

For more details on its effectiveness, as well as the right dose of vitamin C to take, and any possible side effects, see chapter 3.

Zinc: It's Elementary, My Dear Watson

Our bodies need zinc only in very small quantities but must have this element to function properly. If you are deficient in zinc, taking nutritional doses of this mineral will make you healthier overall and might reduce the number of colds you get.

Another way of using zinc is to suck on zinc gluconate or zinc acetate lozenges at the onset of a cold. It seems that zinc can kill viruses directly in the throat and can help shorten the length of time you are sick.

Vitamin C appears to help make colds shorter and less severe.

Before you jump right in and start taking zinc, though, please see chapter 4 and read about how much to take. Too much zinc for too long a time period can be toxic, and it can also upset the balance of other elements needed in your system, such as copper, magnesium, and iron.

Andrographis: Exotic Remedy from the Far East Meets the Common Cold

The common cold is, of course, common to everyone everywhere, so we can learn new methods for treating it by checking out what the folks in other countries do about it. For example, a popular treatment for colds and flus in modern Scandinavia is actually an ancient remedy "borrowed" from India.

A few well-designed double-blind studies that found andrographis effective have recently been published in English. The evidence suggests that andrographis reduces the severity of symptoms and shortens the length of colds—and might actually help prevent them.

Even though andrographis is widely used in Scandinavia for treating colds, its availability in the United States is limited. You can order this herb via the Internet, but you're unlikely to find it in your local pharmacy as yet. For more detail about andrographis, as well as a discussion of possible safety issues involved with using this herb, see chapter 5.

More Treatments to Try for That Cold or Flu

We wish all the herbs and supplements that exist were thoroughly researched so we could have a better idea of what works and what doesn't. Unfortunately, this isn't the case. For a number of reasons, there has been little or no data collected for many such treatments. Of course, this doesn't necessarily mean they don't work—it just means that we don't know for sure whether

they *do* work. See chapter 6 for the information we do have on several other possible cold and flu treatments: elderberry, osha root, yarrow, kudzu, ginger, slippery elm, mullein, marshmallow, arginine, and peppermint.

Evidence suggests that andrographis reduces the severity of symptoms and shortens the length of colds.

Preventing Illness

What's better than a shorter illness? No illness at all! All the treatments we've mentioned so far are geared toward treating colds and flu once you've already begun to feel the symptoms. Some herbs and supplements have been studied for their effectiveness in protecting you from getting sick in the first place.

Ginseng: More Than Just an Energy Booster

Although you may think of ginseng as an herb that gives you energy, an intriguing recent double-blind study suggests that regular use of ginseng may actually stimulate the immune system. Specifically, it may reduce the chance of catching a cold or flu. Echinacea can't do this. Numerous other studies have revealed interesting information about how ginseng may work, but unfortunately, many of them are not the most reliable kind of study. (See chapter 7.)

Adaptogens: For Better Overall Health

Some herbal practitioners have labeled ginseng and certain other plants "adaptogens." An adaptogen is an herb that is said to bring your body into balance, thereby improving your overall resistance to illness as well as other harmful outside influences. While no solid evidence proves that these plants live up to the adaptogen label, quite a bit of evidence suggests that *Panax ginseng* (Asian ginseng) may be effective in improving one's resistance to illness. Another herb often placed in this category is ashwagandha, sometimes called "Indian ginseng."

The medicinal mushroom maitake is also considered an adaptogen. Originally growing wild in the mountains of northeastern Japan and now cultivated by Japanese farmers, it contains chemical components that may stimulate immune system activity. At this time, practitioners who use maitake do so more on the basis of its historic use rather than scientific evidence.

Evidence suggests that *Panax ginseng* (Asian ginseng) may help improve your resistance to illness.

The Brazilian herb suma, the Russian herb rodiola, and another Japanese fungus called reishi mushroom are also said to be adaptogens.

The Chinese herb astragalus is also occasionally classified as an adaptogen. Chinese herbalists have used it for centuries in combination with other herbs for a variety of purposes, including protecting against colds. However, no reliable scientific evidence backs up this use. Again, this does not necessarily mean it doesn't work—only that few studies exist. And again, the studies we have aren't the best kind, which are those that use real, live human beings and are properly designed.

All these potential adaptogen herbs, their traditional uses, research, dosages, and safety information are presented in chapter 7.

Vitamin E and Company: Non-Adaptogens with Preventive Potential

Vitamin E has been very well studied for a variety of the benefits it has to offer, and we may now be able to add one more to its repertoire. A recent double-blind study suggests that vitamin E may offer immune benefits. You'll find the details on vitamin

E's accomplishments in chapter 8, along with information on dosage, safety, and so forth.

In addition to discussing vitamin E, we also revisit the herb andrographis in regard to its potential for preventing colds and flus, as well as a few other treatments that have been studied for cold prevention but with less positive results.

Your Mother Should Know

There is also some good, old-fashioned "mom-like" advice in chapter 9 on what you can do to avoid getting a cold, or how you might treat your symptoms if you do succumb.

What the Doctor Ordered

For more detailed information on the conventional medications you're used to seeing at the drugstore, and those antibiotics you really shouldn't be taking for your viral illness, see chapter 10.

So now you know where to look for some particular information you want. If you want to jump right ahead to something specific, that's fine. If you want a little more information on how we determine what evidence is "strongest," see the following section.

Scientific Method

What constitutes "strong evidence" of a treatment's effectiveness? Well, it's partly a matter of how many studies have been done and whether the results have been positive—that is, suggest that the treatment works. But evidence must be more than that to be considered strong. Determining whether a treatment really works is not as easy as you might think.

The Power of Suggestion: Placebos and Double-Blinding

The main problem is the confusing influence caused by the power of suggestion. If you were given a sugar pill and told it would make you feel better, chances are good that you would feel better. This so-called placebo effect is surprisingly powerful. For some conditions, such as menopausal symptoms or prostate disease, a placebo treatment can essentially make symptoms disappear in as many as 50% of people.[1] While nothing is wrong with healing diseases with placebos (if it can help us feel better, why knock it?), this phenomenon makes it tricky to determine how well a treatment works in itself.

To get around this problem, researchers use the so-called blinded placebo-controlled study. Half the patients involved in the study are given real treatment (the treatment group), while the other half are given phony, or placebo, treatment (the control group), and all patients are kept in the dark (are "blind") about which group they are in. This technique factors out the power of suggestion. If the treatment group does significantly better than the placebo control group, then researchers can conclude that the treatment really works.

It's also important to make sure that the doctor dispensing the pills doesn't know who is in which group. Doctors who are confident that they are giving a real treatment might unintentionally communicate this confidence to patients; this acts as the power of positive suggestion. They also tend to rate the results more optimistically for the group they know is getting a real medication. When both the doctor and the participant are in the dark, the experiment is considered a "double-blind" experiment. This way, the element of suggestion is eliminated. Generally speaking, we can trust only double-blind trials; we must consider the results of other types of studies to be contaminated by the mysterious power of the placebo effect.

While keeping the subjects "blind" is very important, it can also be tricky. For example, the smell and taste of a liquid preparation of echinacea (and some other herbs) is distinctive. Creating a substance that looks and tastes similar but has no active ingredients is difficult. This means that those in the treatment group may know they are taking the real thing and those in the control group may know they are taking a placebo. Similar problems occur in studies of conventional medications. If a treatment causes side effects, participants and physicians may be able to tell whether they are part of the verum (treated) group rather than the placebo (untreated) group. A reliable study will report on efforts to keep the subjects "blind."

Number Crunching

Mark Twain once said that there were three kinds of lies: lies, damn lies, and statistics. We hate to contradict an American hero, but in the research world statistics are a very important way of getting at the truth. One critical concept related to interpreting the results of a study is "statistical significance."

Sometimes you will read that people in the treatment group did better than those in the placebo group but that the results were not statistically significant. This means you cannot assume that the results proved the treatment was effective. Statistical significance is a mathematical technique used to ensure that the apparent improvement seen in the treated group represents a genuine difference, rather than just chance.

Consider the following analogy: Suppose you flip one coin 20 times and end up with 9 heads. Then, you flip a second coin 20 times and count 12 heads. Does this mean that the first coin is less likely to fall with the head side up than the second coin? Or was the difference just due to chance? A special mathematical technique can help answer this question. Similarly, if a group of 20 patients takes echinacea and 9 of them catch a cold, while another group of 20 takes a placebo and 12 of them catch a cold, a mathematical technique can tell us whether this represents a true difference or is just the effect of chance. The bottom line is that when study results look good but aren't statistically significant, they can't be taken any more seriously than the apparent "bias" of the coin that happens to fall heads more often when you flip it a few times.

It's ALIVE! . . . and Human

Here's one more factor to think about when you're examining the evidence. How much do you really have in common with a petri dish full of cells? Or a rat, for that matter?

Studies that use living creatures—people or animals—are called *in vivo* studies. Although studies in animals can give us a lot of information, animals are different from people; therefore, the results don't always transfer. Human studies are, of course, most meaningful to humans.

Other studies, called *in vitro* studies, are performed in test tubes. Researchers may take human cells, grow large populations of them, and then expose them to medicines, toxic substances, or anything else to be studied. Even when these tests use human cells, the cells they study do not function in the whole context of the human body. It is sort of like trying to find out whether children will enjoy playing with a basketball by giving a child isolated in a room a basketball to play with. You won't get the same response you would have if you'd turned a group of kids loose with the ball on a playground where there is a basketball hoop. Similarly, the results of in vitro tests have to be taken as highly preliminary in predicting how the substances tested might behave in the human body.

The reason we discuss the nature of studies at length is that much of the research information presented in this book, while interesting, can't be taken as scientific proof that the treatments are effective, simply due to the questionable quality of the studies. Nonetheless, some of these studies are widely quoted, as if they actually prove something. Understanding these details of research methods will help you understand why the studies aren't as helpful as they could be.

In the following chapters, sections in which we discuss the research in more detail will start with the best studies, the double-blind placebo-controlled studies, because these provide the most meaningful answers to the question: "Will it make you feel better?"

Echinacea: The Most Famous Herb for Colds

E chinacea (pronounced "ek-ih-NAY-sha") is the most famous herbal cold treatment available today. Good evidence shows that, when taken at the onset of a cold or flu, echinacea can reduce the duration and severity of illness. But does it strengthen the immune system when taken long term? Probably not.

Also called purple coneflower, this relative of aster and daisies is a native North American plant that grows wild and in gardens throughout the United States. Echinacea flowers have a large, dark central cone surrounded by daisy-like petals that may be purple, white, yellow, coral, or red, depending on the species.

The word "echinacea" comes from the Greek word "echinos," which means sea urchin or hedgehog. It probably got this name from the prickly spikes found on the flower head (see figure 1). Eight species of echinacea have been identified, but only three are commonly used as medicinal herbs: *E. purpurea*, *E. angustifolia*, and *E. pallida*. Echinacea, like many medicinal plants, is a weed; but it has become popular with gardeners. It is easy to grow from seed, will grow in drought conditions, and even adapts to rocky soil. At the end of its growing season, echinacea produces lots of seeds that will give you an even denser patch of beautiful coneflowers the following year. You can also

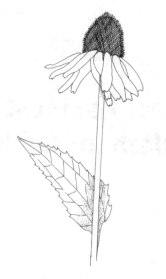

Figure 1. Echinacea purpurea, *also known as purple coneflower*

cultivate echinacea as a perennial by trimming the stalks to a few inches above the ground and letting the plants grow back the following year.

The three medicinal species of echinacea are similar but do have a few notable chemical differences. Each contains different combinations and amounts of the compounds found in echinacea, a unique pattern that gives each species an identifiable chemical fingerprint. Clinical studies have been performed with all three species, sometimes alone and sometimes in combination, however, and it is not clear that one variety is more effective than the others.

What Was Echinacea Used for Historically?

Native Americans have used echinacea medicinally for perhaps thousands of years, long before they introduced the herb to European settlers early in the nineteenth century.

The herb was also used by the Eclectics, physicians who believed in using any method or medicine that might be useful in improving health. Great proponents of botanical medicines, the Eclectics wrote books detailing the medicinal uses of many western plants, including echinacea.[1]

In the late 1800s, echinacea's popularity was given a boost by a flamboyant fellow calling himself Dr. H. C. F. Meyer—though his actual training and background are highly questionable. Meyer promoted an herbal concoction containing echinacea, using techniques reminiscent of religious revival movements. He promoted echinacea so determinedly that the well-respected Lloyd Brothers Pharmacy finally put it to the test themselves and were convinced of the herb's value as a treatment.

By the 1920s, the Lloyd Brothers Pharmacy reported that echinacea was the best-selling product in the history of their company. Echinacea continued to be a very popular cold and flu remedy in the United States until it was displaced by sulfa antibiotics. Ironically, antibiotics are not at all effective for colds and flus, which are usually viral infections untouched by antibiotics, while echinacea *does* appear to be beneficial in such cases.

Echinacea Today: Traditional Herb Meets Twentieth-Century Science

Although physicians in the United States and Canada eventually stopped using herbal remedies in general, including echinacea, the herb didn't fall out of favor in Europe. A mounting body of scientific evidence led Germany, in 1992, to authorize the use of echinacea root extracts for "the supportive treatment of flu-like infections" and echinacea juice for "supportive treatment of recurrent infections of the upper respiratory tract and lower urinary tract."[2] In Germany today, at least 300 products on the market contain echinacea, and the herb is the most commonly prescribed treatment for the common cold.

In the United States, however, patients often request antibiotics for colds (and physicians too frequently prescribe them), despite the fact that antibiotics are ineffective against viruses. For more information on the dangers of using antibiotics in this

Accidental Popularity

The Native Americans in the plains region used *E. angustifolia* more than any other medicinal plant. Because of this, Europeans who settled in North America were most familiar with this variety, so European herbal product manufacturers originally concentrated on acquiring *E. angustifolia*. During a period when American sources did not meet the European demand, a German pharmaceutical company mistakenly bought seeds of *E. purpurea* and grew them for medicinal use. This case of mistaken identity is the primary reason *E. purpurea* has become the main type of echinacea we use today.

inappropriate way, see chapter 10, which will cover conventional treatment.

That old saying, "A cold lasts 7 days, but if you take care of yourself, you can get over it in a week," was based on the knowledge that conventional treatment can't help a cold—but whoever said it first may not have known about echinacea. An ever-increasing amount of scientific evidence shows that echinacea can help you get over a cold significantly faster. The herb can also make the symptoms of your cold milder and might help you "abort" a cold that has just started. However, contrary to what you may have read, daily use of echinacea throughout the winter probably won't stop you from getting sick.

The Clinical Studies

The studies that have most relevance are those that test the therapy on real, live humans to see whether it works. Many such clinical studies have focused on echinacea, and most come from Germany, where echinacea is a commonly prescribed medicine.

By 1999, at least 29 controlled clinical studies of the effects of echinacea had been completed, 14 of which were double blind.[3-6] Most of this research examined echinacea with respect to upper respiratory tract infections, which means illnesses involving the nose, throat, and bronchi. Colds and flus are upper respiratory tract infections. All together, these studies make a relatively good case that echinacea in its various forms can reduce the number of days of sickness and make cold and flu symptoms milder. However, the evidence that echinacea can actually *prevent* colds is weak.

Help Wanted: Only Snotty People Need Apply

In Uppsala, Sweden, during the fall of 1996, a group of researchers ran an ad in the newspaper seeking people who would be willing to participate in a study on using echinacea if they happened to catch a cold or flu. Two hundred forty-six responders came down with colds during the study period. On a random basis, each participant was selected to receive either a placebo or one of three types of tablets made from *E. purpurea*. The first type of tablet contained 6.78 mg of crude extract made from 95% herbs (leaves, stems, and flowers) and 5% roots; the second was of the same formula at a higher concentration of 48.27 mg; and the third was made only from the roots of the plant, at 29.60 mg.

At the first onset of symptoms, participants took two of whichever kind of tablets they had been assigned 3 times daily for 7 days (or until they felt well, whichever came first). They kept diaries of their symptoms and were also examined by the investigators three times during their illness. Neither the participants nor the people examining them knew which kind of tablets they were taking—making it a double-blind study.

The results seen with both of the formulas containing echinacea leaf, stem, and flower were quite good.

Echinacea may help you get over a cold significantly faster.

Treatment was rated as effective by about 60% of physicians and at a slightly higher rate by the participants themselves. (Technically, this was the result using an "intention to treat analysis," a method that takes into account participants who dropped out of the study. If you look at everyone who completed the study, the percentages are even higher, but for technical reasons that's cheating.) The fact that there was little difference in improvement between the low and high concentrations of this formula suggests that the lower dose is sufficient; more isn't better.

Interestingly, the root-only formula didn't work at all in this study. We might guess from this that some of the effective ingredients of *E. purpurea* are more concentrated in the aboveground portions of the plant.

However, another double-blind placebo-controlled study that followed 180 people given an alcohol extract of *E. purpurea* roots did find positive results.[7] The group taking a low dose of the root extract did not show significant improvements when compared to the placebo group. However, the group taking a higher dose did show a statistically significant improvement in severity and duration of cold symptoms. Apparently, *E. purpurea* roots do work; you just need to take enough.

Other species of echinacea have been found to work too. A double-blind placebo-controlled study using *E. pallida* followed 160 adults with a recent onset of an upper respiratory infection (cold, flu, or other causes). Patients were given *E. pallida* or a placebo for 10 days. The results showed a statistically significant reduction in the duration of illness, from 13 days in the placebo group to about 9.5 days in the treated group.

Positive results were also seen in a double-blind placebo-controlled study of 100 people with acute upper respiratory infections (URIs) given either a placebo or a combination product that was mostly *E. angustifolia*.[8]

Putting it all together, it appears from these studies that all three types of echinacea can shorten the duration of colds and improve cold symptoms. You really can treat a cold to make it go away faster.

Aborting Colds

The studies described suggest that echinacea may help reduce the symptoms of colds. But what about avoiding them altogether? Can echinacea help with that? The ambiguous answer: yes and no.

On the positive side, results of one study suggested that echinacea can sometimes stop a cold that is just starting. In this study, 120 people were given *E. purpurea* or a placebo as soon as they started showing signs of getting a cold. This study was double blinded and lasted a total of 10 days after each person started taking either the echinacea or the placebo. Participants took either echinacea or the placebo at a dose of 20 drops every 2 hours for 1 day, then 20 drops 3 times per day for 9 more days.

Echinacea does not appear to be useful for preventing colds.

Fewer people in the echinacea group felt that their initial symptoms actually developed into "real" colds (40% of those taking echinacea versus 60% taking the placebo actually became ill). This suggests that taking echinacea can sometimes "abort" a cold in its early phases.

Not surprisingly, based on what other studies have shown, echinacea also provided benefits for those who did become ill. But stopping a cold from starting is even better than making it go away faster!

Some people try to use echinacea in another way. They take it regularly throughout cold season in hopes of not getting a cold at all. However, studies that have evaluated whether this method works have not yielded very promising results. Suffice it to say for now that echinacea is better used right at the onset of a cold to reduce its severity and duration or, with luck, to nip it in the bud; it is not very effective, if at all, as a long-term preventive treatment. For more details on the studies, and for information on herbs for cold and flu prevention, see chapter 7.

Not Just for Colds and Flus

Most clinical use of echinacea focuses on colds and flus, but this herb has been used for other illnesses too. However, the scientific evidence for these conditions is not strong.

For example, studies have examined echinacea's ability to fight the common yeast *Candida albicans,* which can cause thrush and vaginal yeast infections. One clinical study found that echinacea can improve the effectiveness of conventional antifungal medications.[9] Unfortunately, because the study was not blinded, it is unclear how much of the outcome was due to the power of suggestion.

Echinacea has also been studied for its wound-healing ability. Several studies have found that echinacea can decrease inflammation in animals and promote wound healing.[10-14] However, none of these studies meets current scientific standards, so they can't be viewed as proof that echinacea helps heal wounds.

How Does Echinacea Work?

So how does echinacea produce its documented benefits in cases of cold or flu? We might as well admit this right up front: No one really knows. Of course, that will never stop scientists from making educated guesses.

What most researchers believe is that echinacea increases what is called *cell-mediated immunity.* This is the part of the immune system involving T-lymphocytes—specialized cells designed to recognize and glom onto just one certain type of invader. They also begin to make copies of themselves once they've spotted their quarry, as well as to release chemicals that act as a rallying cry to the rest of your immune system. You'll only have T-lymphocytes present in your body for antigens to which you've been exposed. Their presence is what keeps you from getting certain kinds of diseases—like mumps or measles—more than once.

Doctors can test this type of immunity using an injection under the skin. If you've been exposed to either the real disease or a vaccine, you should show a reaction to this test. If you know you've been exposed, but you don't react, it may be that your immune system is simply "sleepy." (The scientific name for this immune laziness is "anergy.")

The Legend of the "Strengthened" Immune System

Many people who talk about echinacea say that it strengthens the immune system. Unfortunately, no scientific evidence supports this theory. Among other possible explanations, it is at least as likely that echinacea simply stimulates the immune system into increased action, perhaps by acting as a "threat." Such stimulation is a far cry from "strengthening" and might not always be good for you. This is the reason echinacea is not recommended in autoimmune diseases.

In one study, echinacea extracts were found to "wake up" the immune system and increase the reaction in tests of cell-mediated immunity.[15] This distinctly suggests that echinacea is an immune stimulant.

Additional studies have examined echinacea's ability to affect the activity of immune cells. These laboratory studies are interesting, and many show that echinacea can stimulate the immune system. However, they have to be taken with a grain of salt, as measures of immune cell activity notoriously say very little about real-life resistance to illness.

One study found that both injected and oral administration of echinacea causes an increase in *phagocytosis*, the swallowing of foreign bodies, by certain immune cells.[16] In this study, phagocytosis increased while echinacea was administered and returned to normal within a few days after echinacea was stopped.

Animal and test tube studies have also found evidence that echinacea increases immune cell activity.[17–23] Unfortunately, an increase in measured levels of cell activity may or may not translate into any meaningful effect on immunity as a whole. A good analogy might be when a certain football coach gets his players to run faster and jump up and down more vigorously in practice. This may be a good sign, but it doesn't necessarily translate into success on the game field. Echinacea's measured effects on immune cells may or may not have anything to do with how it works.

Finally, the effects of echinacea are often described as "strengthening the immune system." Actually, it is at least as likely that echinacea merely stimulates the immune system into a short-term burst of increased activity. It may do so by acting like a "threat" to which the body responds by calling out the immune system's equivalent of the National Guard. The immune cells activated to fight echinacea may then go on to fight whatever virus is present at the same time.

Some manufacturers advocate using the pressed juices of the plant, rather than an extraction.

This explanation fits with the observed results in studies. If echinacea strengthened immunity, you'd think that taking it long term would help prevent colds. But as we shall see in chapter 7, it doesn't work that way. Rather, echinacea seems to function best as a *short-term* treatment. One could say that keeping the National Guard on alert all the time would eventually decrease its effectiveness. Other treatments, such as ginseng, are better candidates as immune strengtheners (see chapter 7 for more information).

Immune stimulation isn't the only possibility. It could be that echinacea merely reduces symptoms. If your symptoms are reduced, you'll *seem* to get over a cold faster because once the symptoms go below a certain point, an effective symptom reducer might make them appear to have disappeared entirely.

What Part of Echinacea Is Responsible for Its Effects?

Echinacea contains several components that produce varying effects, both in animals (including humans) and in cells in test tubes. Some components are found in the roots; some exist only in the flowers or stems. However, we don't know which are the most important.

If we knew which components were most important, this information could prove valuable when you make or buy medicinal extracts of echinacea. For instance, some components of

The Tongue-Tingle Test

E pallida's chemical components are not dramatically different from those of *E. purpurea*, except that *E. pallida* does not contain cichoric acid or alkylamides.[33–36] Alkylamides are what make your tongue tingle after you take liquid echinacea. While we don't know whether alkylamides are one of the active ingredients, their presence (or absence) definitely helps you identify species. If you've purchased a liquid identified as *E. angustifolia* or *E. purpurea* and your tongue doesn't tingle when you take it, you have either *E. pallida* or something that isn't echinacea at all.

echinacea are water-soluble and some are alcohol-soluble. Predictably, an alcohol extract will have mostly alcohol-soluble components and very few water-soluble ones, while the reverse is true when you make an infusion or "tea." However, since we don't know which components matter most, it's hard to make a clear recommendation as to which form of echinacea is best to make or buy. Some manufacturers advocate using the pressed juices of the plant, rather than an extraction, in order to get nearly all possible ingredients.

Some of echinacea's known components have labels you're probably not familiar with: caffeic acids, cichoric acid, echinacoside, caffeic acid, and cynarine; flavonoids; immunostimulatory polysaccharides; polyacetylenes; alkylamides; isobutylamides; alkaloids; and essential oils.[24–27] Researchers have studied many of these components in an attempt to understand what makes echinacea work.

Candidates so far nominated for active ingredient(s) include various polysaccharides (especially arabinogalactan), cichoric acid, and certain polyacetylenes and isobutylamides.[28–32]

However, despite quite a number of laboratory studies, the dispute remains unsettled.

Dosage

Even if we don't know *how* it works, the evidence is pretty good that echinacea does work. However, you need to use it properly.

Echinacea is usually taken at the first sign of a cold and continued for 7 to 14 days. The typical dosage of echinacea powdered extract is 300 mg 3 times a day. Alcohol tincture (1:5) is usually taken at a dosage of 3 to 4 ml 3 times daily, echinacea juice at a dosage of 2 to 3 ml 3 times daily, and whole dried root at 1 to 2 g 3 times daily. Certain proprietary formulas may require different dosing, so read the label carefully.

We don't really know which of the many forms of echinacea is best. At the present time, it's also difficult to recommend one of the three species of echinacea—*purpurea, angustifolia,* or *pallida.* All seem to work. However, regardless of species, many herbalists feel that it is important the herb contacts the back of the throat, reasoning that it stimulates the lymph glands there.

The three species of echinacea— *purpurea, angusti- folia,* or *pallida*— all seem to work.

Goldenseal is frequently combined with echinacea in preparations meant to be taken at the first sign of a cold. However, no real evidence suggests that oral goldenseal stimulates immunity or helps colds. Furthermore, traditional herbalists did not use it in this way.[37]

Safety Issues

Echinacea appears to be safe. Even when taken in very high doses, it has not been found to cause any toxic effects.[38,39] Reported side effects are also uncommon and usually limited to minor gastrointestinal symptoms, increased urination, and mild allergic reactions.[40]

Studies dating back to the 1950s suggest that injected echinacea is safe in children. Does this mean that present-day oral echinacea products are safe for children? Quite likely, but we can't guarantee it.

Commission E, which is Germany's version of the United States's FDA, warns against using echinacea in cases of auto-immune disorders such as multiple sclerosis, lupus, and rheumatoid arthritis, as well as tuberculosis or leukocytosis. There are also rumors that echinacea should not be used by people with AIDS. These warnings are theoretical, based on fears that echinacea might actually activate immunity in the wrong way. While they are sensible precautions, at the present time no evidence indicates that echinacea use has actually harmed anyone with these diseases.

The Commission E monograph on echinacea—an informative paper summarizing what is known about the plant—also recommends against using echinacea for more than 8 weeks. The safety of echinacea in young children, pregnant or nursing women, or those with severe liver or kidney disease has not been established. There are no known drug interactions.

Other Herbal Remedies

Echinacea is probably the best known, and best researched, of the herbal remedies and supplements used for flus and colds; but it is far from being the only one. Read on to find more information on the efficacy of vitamin C, zinc, andrographis, and many more natural remedies for your miseries.

Visit Us at TNP.com

World Explorers and Nobel Prize Winners: The History of a Vitamin

Did you ever wonder why all the swashbuckling pirates and common sailors in those old movies were bow-legged and toothless? In fact, this cinematic representation reflects a stylized version of scurvy and its so-called "scorbutic symptoms"— nonhealing wounds, bleeding gums, loss of teeth, bruising, and overall weakness. Sudden death following physical exertion was also considered a classic symptom.

Although vitamin C itself would not be discovered for over a century, some eighteenth-century British captains had already come to recognize that citrus fruit could keep their crews free of the dread sailors' disease. In 1747, the Scottish physician James Lind tested this theory using one of history's first controlled experiments. He treated 12 scorbutic seaman with six

Orange juice is the quintessential source of vitamin C, but many vegetables are richer sources.

different diets. Citrus fruit was found to be so effective in causing the symptoms to abate that he ended his study and treated the rest of the patients thus, curing them all.

In making this discovery, James Lind had reinvented a wheel previously known to the Phoenicians, seagoing explorers from Africa about 2,000 years earlier. But it would be a half-century before the British Admiralty took heed. In 1796, the British navy mandated (and paid for) carrying vitamin C–containing lemon and lime juice on board their ships. The British "limeys," as they became known for this custom, no longer lost half or more of their crew to scurvy on long voyages, and quickly came to rule the seas.

We now know that scurvy is nothing more or less than vitamin C deficiency. One of this vitamin's main functions is helping the body manufacture collagen, a key protein in numerous tissues, including skin, the lining of blood vessels, and the valves of the heart. Without it, these tissues weaken, leading to the classic symptoms of scurvy.

Though vitamin C thus changed the course of seafaring history, it wasn't identified in its pure form until 1928. During that year, Hungarian researcher Albert Szent-Gyorgyi isolated the active ingredient from oranges and cabbages, and called it the "anti-scorbutic principle," or ascorbic acid for short. He received the Nobel Prize for his discovery. As certain other dietary elements were discovered to be essential nutrients, they were christened "vitamins" and assigned a letter based on the order in which they were identified. (Some were later determined not to be essential after all, hence the gaps between vitamin E and K.)

Vitamin C really made headlines in the 1960s, when two-time Nobel Prize winner Dr. Linus Pauling claimed that vitamin C could effectively treat both cancer and the common cold. This announcement stirred up much controversy . . . and also inspired a great deal of scientific research.

Vitamin C and Colds

As the most famous of all natural treatments for colds, vitamin C has been subjected to irresponsible hype from both proponents and opponents. Enthusiasts claim that if you take vitamin C daily, you will never get sick, while enemies of the treatment insist that vitamin C offers no benefit at all. There's nothing like creating a well-publicized stir in the scientific community to generate funds for research, and we owe much of what we know about vitamin C to Dr. Pauling. Innumerable researchers were motivated to try to either prove or disprove his claims.

Research indicates that vitamin C supplements can significantly reduce symptoms of colds.

A cool-headed evaluation of the research indicates that vitamin C supplements can significantly reduce symptoms of colds and help you get over a cold slightly faster.[1,2] However, a misleading review article published in the 1970s stated that vitamin C had no real effect at all.[3] After this article was published, many physicians adopted a negative attitude toward vitamin C. But a close look at the data shows that the article's conclusions were biased. The reviewer included studies in which subjects took as little as 25 mg of vitamin C daily—less than what you'd get in half an orange.[4] You clearly need more vitamin C than that if you want to see any benefits. (More information on the right dose to use comes later in this chapter.)

Vitamin C may also prevent some colds, though the data is not overwhelmingly positive.

In fact, in 11 studies during which participants took 1,000 mg or more vitamin C daily, symptom severity was reduced by 40%, and the average length of colds was shortened by a day. Now granted, it's not easy to think about your own cold in terms of numbers. What does a 40% reduction in symptoms feel like? Using 60 tissues instead of 100? Actually, some specific improvements reported included less sore throat pain; less feverishness, aching, and chills; and reduced nasal stuffiness. Getting up to full speed in 6 rather than 7 days is less impressive, but still means something.

Does vitamin C work as well for flus as it does for colds? We don't know. The question has not been well studied.

Vitamin C may also prevent some colds, though the data is not overwhelmingly positive. The results of numerous studies suggest that regular use of vitamin C can slightly reduce the number of colds you get each year, by perhaps 20%.[5] One particular type of cold may respond better than others: the respiratory infection that can follow endurance exercise. Also, individuals who are significantly deficient in vitamin C will find they stay healthier if they make sure to get enough. For more details on vitamin C for prevention, see chapter 8.

How Does Vitamin C Work?

There are several theories about how vitamin C may be acting within our bodies to combat our cold symptoms. Of course, no one is certain, but researchers are able to make some pretty well educated guesses by observing some of the biochemical changes that occur in our cells.

Vitamin C is an antioxidant. This means it neutralizes certain harmful molecules known as free radicals that are generated by the chemical reactions going on in our bodies. When the body puts on a defense against viruses and bacteria, it creates a larger-than-usual number of these damaging molecules. These may unintentionally cause some of the classic cold symptoms. One theory is that vitamin C may be relieving some of our cold symptoms by "defusing" these free radicals.[6]

Also, some evidence from laboratory studies suggests that neutrophils, one of our bodies' defense cells, are more effective when higher levels of vitamin C are available to them. This mechanism would not explain the entire effect of the vitamin on cold symptoms (neutrophils don't fight viruses), but could contribute some benefit for secondary bacterial infections. Another theory sometimes advanced is that vitamin C helps colds by acting as a sort of natural antihistamine. However, since regular antihistamines do little for colds or flus, this explanation doesn't make much sense.

A final, but even less likely, possibility is that the vitamin is assisting in a chemical reaction that inactivates viruses directly. This is unlikely because, to do so, vitamin C would have to play a role essentially opposite of what it is best known for doing— being an antioxidant. However, some researchers have speculated that under certain conditions, this could be possible.

Researchers will undoubtedly be kept busy for a long time trying to piece together the entire puzzle. For now, we have enough clinical studies to feel fairly certain that vitamin C does work, even if we don't know precisely how.

Dosage

The current U.S. Recommended Dietary Allowances (RDA) for vitamin C are shown in the sidebar on page 37. If you consume the recommended amount of vitamin C, you would be fairly certain to avoid any overt problems due to a vitamin C deficiency, such as scurvy.

Scurvy is now a rarity in the developed world. However, a more subtle deficiency of vitamin C is fairly common, especially among hospital patients.[7-11] Also, aspirin, other anti-inflammatory drugs, corticosteroids, and tetracycline-family antibiotics might lower body levels of vitamin C.[12-14]

Furthermore, even if current recommended daily allowances of vitamin C are enough to prevent scurvy, new recommendations under consideration may raise the recommended intake. The very concept of the RDA is changing. Researchers are now trying to identify the proper dose of vitamins to promote optimal health, rather than just to avoid symptoms of deficiency. Based on this principle, adults may soon be advised to consume about 200 mg of vitamin C daily.

If you eat plenty of fruits and vegetables, you may be meeting your RDA without taking vitamin C in pill form. One great advantage of getting vitamin C from foods rather than from supplements is that you will get many other healthy nutrients at the same time, such as bioflavonoids and carotenes. However, vitamin C in food is partially destroyed by cooking and exposure to air, so for maximum nutritional benefit, you might want to try freshly made salads rather than dishes that require a lot of cooking.

Keep in mind that many of the positive clinical studies mentioned above involved far more than even the new RDA proposal: 1,000 mg (1 g) per day. Linus Pauling and his followers sometimes went further and recommended taking vitamin C doses as high as 20 to 30 g (20,000 to 30,000 mg) daily. The idea is that you should take as much vitamin C as you can, up to 30,000 mg daily, cutting back only when you start to develop stomach cramps and diarrhea.

U.S. Recommended Dietary Allowance for Vitamin C

Infants under 6 months	30 mg
Infants 6 to 12 months	35 mg
Children 1 to 3 years	40 mg
Children 4 to 10 years	45 mg
Children 11 to 14 years	50 mg
Adults (and teenagers 15 years and older)	60 mg
Pregnant women	70 mg
Nursing women	90 to 95 mg

This recommendation is based less on evidence that such huge doses of vitamin C are good for you, as on evangelistic enthusiasm.

However, reasonably impressive evidence suggests that there are diminishing returns with increasing vitamin C intake. It turns out that if you consume more than 200 mg daily (researchers have tested up to 2,500 mg), your kidneys begin to excrete the excess at a steadily increasing rate, matching the increased dose. At the same time, your digestive tract also stops absorbing it well. The net effect may be that you're doing no more than giving your digestive tract and kidneys a vitamin C bath when you take more than the 200 mg daily dosage; your blood level of vitamin C won't increase.

Taking 400 to 1,000 mg of vitamin C in multiple daily doses likely provides the most vitamin C possible.

However, this research contains some potential flaws. Most notably, the evidence presented doesn't rule out the possibility that dividing up your vitamin C dosage into several daily doses might increase blood levels. Furthermore, it is possible that vitamin C levels in the tissues continue to increase to some extent.

So how much should you take? Based on the evidence, it is likely that taking 400 to 1,000 mg of vitamin C each day divided into two or more daily doses will give you the maximum possible body levels of vitamin C. However, if you really want to take 500 mg 6 times a day for the first week or two of your cold, it's unlikely to cause you harm. Not only that, if you purchase vitamin C in lozenge form, you may enjoy the throat-soothing effect.

Safety Issues

Vitamin C is generally recognized as safe when taken at dosages up to 500 mg daily,[15] and even enormous doses should be quite safe when taken short term for colds. Media reports that vitamin C can cause DNA damage were based on an exaggerated interpretation of a fairly theoretical finding.[16]

However, high-dose or long-term vitamin C usage presents possible problems, especially for people with certain fairly rare medical conditions.

If you take more than 1,000 to 2,000 mg of vitamin C daily, you may develop diarrhea. This side effect usually goes away with continued use of vitamin C; but if you want to take this much vitamin C, you should cut down your dosage for a while, and then build up again gradually.

High-dose vitamin C can cause copper deficiency and excessive iron absorption. There is also reason to believe that long-term vitamin C treatment might increase the risk of kidney stones in certain people.[17,18] Actually, in a large-scale study, the people who took the most vitamin C (over 1,500 mg daily) showed a *lower* risk of kidney stones than those taking the least amounts.[19,20] Nonetheless, to be on the safe side, individuals with a history of kidney stones, or who are known to have a defect in vitamin C or oxalate metabolism, should probably restrict vitamin C intake to approximately 100 mg daily.[21]

If you have glucose-6-phosphate dehydrogenase deficiency (a genetic defect resulting in anemia), iron overload, kidney failure, or a history of intestinal surgery, you should use vitamin C only under medical supervision.

According to early reports, high-dose vitamin C might reduce the blood-thinning effects of Coumadin (warfarin) and heparin,[22,23] but subsequent research has failed to corroborate this.[24]

The maximum safe dosages of vitamin C for young children, pregnant or nursing women, or those with severe liver or kidney disease have not been determined.

Beyond Colds: Vitamin C's Other Possible Benefits

After Linus Pauling started the craze, vitamin C was touted as a possible remedy for almost every illness you can imagine. Cancer prevention and treatment, heart disease prevention, hypertension, asthma, low sperm count, bedsores, Alzheimer's disease, diabetes, hepatitis, herpes, insomnia, osteoarthritis, Parkinson's disease, periodontal disease, preeclampsia, rheumatoid arthritis, ulcers, allergies, general antioxidant, bladder infections, menopausal symptoms, migraine headaches, and nausea are only a few of the conditions for which vitamin C was recommended.

You might have noticed that we didn't say vitamin C successfully treats all these conditions. Research has explored some of these possible medicinal uses of vitamin C, but not all of them. And of the uses studied, little if any benefit was found in most cases.

Two health conditions for which vitamin C supplements seem to have some real potential include prevention of cataracts and macular degeneration.[25-30] For more information on these possibilities, see Prima Health's *The Natural Pharmacist: Natural Treatments for Diabetes* and *The Natural Pharmacist: The Natural Health Bible* chapter entitled "Cataracts."

Small double-blind studies suggest that vitamin C may also be able to speed recovery from bedsores,[31] increase sperm count,[32] and reduce asthma symptoms.[33] Vitamin C may modestly reduce blood pressure as well.[34,35] However, most of the studies regarding blood pressure were not of the double-blind variety, so the results can't be taken as fully reliable. Indeed, one double-blind study pertaining to blood pressure found *no* difference between vitamin C and a placebo.[36]

Eating a diet rich in vitamin C appears to reduce the risks of cancer and heart disease, and to slow the progression of osteo-arthritis;[37,38] however, supplemental vitamin C hasn't been found to provide the same benefits. As noted earlier, foods containing vitamin C also contain many other healthful ingredients (such as bioflavonoids and carotenes), and it's not clear which of these ingredients are responsible. Perhaps the entire combination is required.

Cancer treatment is one of the more controversial proposed uses of vitamin C. Two studies have shown high doses of vitamin C supplement to prolong the lives of terminal cancer patients;[39,40] however, other studies have found no benefit of vitamin C in cancer treatment.[41,42] At the present time, vitamin C cannot be regarded as a proven treatment for cancer. It is also controversial whether *any* antioxidants should be taken during cancer chemotherapy. Cancer patients should talk with their oncologists about the wisdom of using any supplements while receiving chemotherapeutic drugs.

As for the rest of the problems mentioned, there simply isn't scientific data to support (or refute) the usefulness of vitamin C.

Zinc for Colds and Flus

Z inc is an important element that is found in every cell in the body. More than 300 enzymes in the body need zinc in order to function properly. In case that doesn't impress you, you should know that without enzymes, most of the chemical reactions that keep us alive would not be able to occur. We need zinc for wound healing, for storing and releasing insulin, and for proper immune function, to name only a few of its uses.

Severe zinc deficiency can cause a major loss of immune function, and mild zinc deficiency might impair immunity slightly. For this reason, making sure to get enough zinc may help keep you from catching colds or other infections. For more information about the preventive aspect of zinc, see chapter 8.

Here we discuss a completely different use of zinc: its role as a virus killer. Rather than taking a zinc supplement to keep your body stores of zinc topped off, you can also take high doses of zinc in lozenge form at the first sign of cold symptoms. Evidence suggests that when used this way, zinc directly fights viruses in the throat, reducing your symptoms and helping you get better faster. The results can be impressive.

Colds: Scientific Evidence of Zinc's Usefulness

Good evidence suggests that if you take the right type of zinc lozenge every 2 hours at the beginning of a cold, you will recover significantly more quickly.[1] Long-term zinc supplementation at nutritional doses may also reduce the chance of getting sick, but probably only if you are deficient in zinc to begin with.[2]

Numerous studies have evaluated the effects of zinc lozenges for colds. The findings suggest that zinc lozenges can significantly improve cold symptoms, as long as the right form of zinc is used (zinc gluconate or acetate, with the right kind of flavorings).[3–5]

For example, a randomized, double-blind study involving 100 hospital employees found that zinc gluconate lozenges markedly decreased the severity and duration of the common cold.[6] Half of the participants used lozenges with 13.3 mg of zinc gluconate every 2 hours (while they were awake) for the duration of their colds. The other half did the same thing with placebo lozenges.

Severe zinc deficiency can cause a major loss of immune function; mild zinc deficiency might impair immunity.

The treated group had statistically significant reductions in cough, headache, hoarseness, nasal congestion, runny nose, and sore throat (see figure 2). In addition, their colds lasted an average of 4.4 days, remarkably less than the 7.6 days' duration of colds for the placebo group. However, zinc did not help fever, muscle aches, scratchy throat, and sneezing. The only side effect noted was mild nausea.

Good results have been seen in several other double-blind studies involving zinc gluconate.[7,8] Although a few other studies seemed at first glance to find no benefit, a close review of the evidence showed that these studies used forms of zinc lozenges that did not release virus-killing zinc ions into the throat. Laws

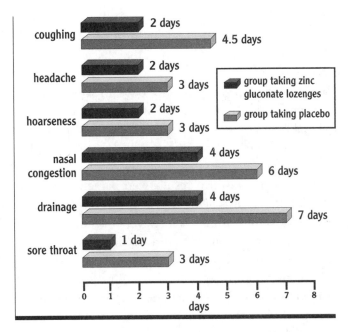

Figure 2. *Double-blind study shows zinc lozenges reduced the number of days participants experienced cold symptoms*

of chemistry dictate how zinc ions are released, and it turns out that only some types of zinc can release the right ions. To be of any benefit, the ions must have a positive charge. Some studies used forms of zinc that released negatively charged ions instead, and it was found that the duration of the colds for those in the treatment group actually increased! Both the chemical form of zinc used and the types of sweeteners added to the lozenges play a role.

One study used one of the "right" forms of zinc, zinc gluconate, but did not find benefits.[9] In this case, children in grades 1 through 6 were given 10 mg of zinc gluconate 5 times per day, and children in grades 7 through 12 were given 10 mg 6 times per day. Zinc did not reduce the duration or severity of colds in these children. The study authors offered several possible explanations for this failure, including that the dose may have been too low, or that the cherry oil used to flavor the lozenges might have interfered with the zinc ions (a reasonable possibility, considering that many other flavorings have been found to interfere).

Zinc acetate lozenges were also found to significantly reduce the duration of cold symptoms in a double-blind placebo-controlled clinical trial.[10] Of the 101 participants who completed the study, 52 took lozenges containing 9 mg of zinc, while 49 took a placebo.

You may have noticed that the doses of zinc gluconate used in studies that had positive results were larger. But laboratory studies have found that all of the zinc in zinc acetate is released as ions in a solution with the same level of acidity as your body, whereas with zinc gluconate, only a fraction (about 30%) of the zinc becomes ions. If this is also true in our bodies—and it probably is—then lower doses of zinc acetate should be needed.

Another plus for the zinc acetate was that no one participating in the study noticed a bitter taste, a complaint heard in most of the studies using zinc gluconate. However, a few people participating in the zinc acetate reported a metallic aftertaste or a chalky taste.

An additional interesting bit of data was collected in this study. The cold sufferers were all tested for the presence of allergies to a wide variety of substances. For the portion of the treatment and placebo groups who tested positive for allergies, the difference in recovery time was even more pronounced, which may suggest that zinc could be useful in treating allergy symptoms as well as colds.

Putting all the evidence together, properly chosen zinc lozenges may be beneficial for colds when started within 48 hours of the onset and used regularly, but further research is necessary to iron out the contradictory reports.[11,12]

How Does Zinc Work?

Several theories about how zinc helps us fight off colds have been proposed, based on studies done in laboratories.[13,14] No one is certain that zinc works the same way in the human body as it did in a test tube, but it's quite possible that it does.

Zinc has been found, in the test tube at least, to prevent rhinoviruses, herpes simplex virus, and Coxsackie virus (all common causes of colds) from manufacturing proteins. If they can't make the proteins, they can't build more virus particles.

Another observation is that zinc may effectively block the "doorways" these virus particles use to get into the cells that line your nose and throat. If they can't get in, they can't breed (remember, viruses have no machinery of their own to reproduce themselves—they have to borrow yours). One way zinc has been found to do this is by binding to the same receptors to which the virus particles would bind.

Zinc has been found, in the test tube, to prevent cold viruses from manufacturing proteins.

Another method by which zinc may block these "doorways" is by more generally making the cells less permeable; zinc acts as an astringent in these cases, meaning it just generally tightens things up and stabilizes the cell membrane. This tightening up of the membrane may also limit the amount of histamine released by your cells, which would have an effect similar to that of taking an antihistamine.

Zinc ions added to cell cultures were found to cause the cells to produce interferon, a protein that our immune system makes to help fight off viruses. Interferon acts as a messenger to other cells in the body, cueing them to make antiviral proteins and T-cells. Some of our cells have been found to release zinc ions in response to both viral infections and allergens, so we may be simply bolstering our own natural defense system—providing more little "soldiers" to beef up the troops—by taking zinc.

Last, but perhaps not least, zinc is known to have antibacterial properties, and its presence in your mouth and throat may

Zinc: Dietary Supplement vs. Cold Therapy

You can use a vitamin or mineral in two different ways: as a dietary supplement or as a therapeutic substance. When you use zinc as a dietary supplement, you're ensuring that your body has an adequate level of zinc to maintain normal health and function. When you use zinc as a therapeutic substance—essentially, as a medicine—you're using it to combat a disease.

A major difference between supplemental and therapeutic use of zinc is in the amount taken, and the duration of use. Specifically, an adult usually needs about 12 to 15 mg per day of zinc for normal function (see chapter 8 for more information on using zinc as a supplement). When used to treat colds, zinc is taken at much higher doses than are needed for everyday physical maintenance, but only for a short

help prevent secondary bacterial infections. Specifically, it has been found to inhibit growth of streptococci (the perpetrators of "strep throat") and actinomyces when added to toothpaste.

We still need to find out more about how zinc really works in our bodies; for now, the clinical evidence is fairly good that the right kind of zinc lozenges can probably lessen some of your symptoms and shorten your cold by a couple of days.

Dosage

You can use zinc in either of two ways: in a low dose for nutritional purposes, or at a high dose during the first week or so of a cold. Here we discuss the high-dose, short-term usage of zinc.

The following dosages are expressed in terms of "elemental zinc." This is the amount of zinc actually present in a zinc compound such as zinc gluconate.

For treatment of colds, the usual dosage of zinc is 13.3 to 23 mg of elemental zinc in the form of zinc gluconate; 13.3 mg is the lowest dose found effective in clinical trials. A slightly time. You might take as much as 23 mg of zinc every 1½ to 2 hours for a week or so, until the symptoms abate—far more than your body normally requires.

Another difference is that the goal in cold treatment is to have the zinc contact your throat directly by dissolving lozenges in your mouth. That way, the zinc goes directly to the infected cells of your upper respiratory tract rather than being absorbed through your digestive tract.

Therapeutic doses of zinc are not recommended for a treatment period longer than 2 weeks (see Safety Issues, page 48), but using zinc for treatment of colds according to these methods has been found to be safe, and in many cases effective.

lower dose of 9 mg of elemental zinc as zinc acetate was found effective in the clinical study mentioned on page 42, in the section "Colds: Scientific Evidence of Zinc's Usefulness," but we don't have enough evidence to know whether this is the optimum dose. We do know that this amount was safe, and that it appeared to work.

Lozenges should be dissolved in the mouth every 2 hours until cold symptoms have disappeared, but should be taken for no longer than 2 weeks. There is no evidence that taking more will increase effectiveness.

Zinc lozenges work best when started as soon as possible after the onset of a cold. The lozenge must be dissolved in your mouth because the zinc ions are absorbed directly into the virus-infected cells of your throat.

Zinc lozenges are usually sweetened or otherwise flavored to disguise their taste, but acidic additives like citrate may bind the zinc ions in your mouth and make it impossible for them to kill the viruses in your throat. Sweet carbohydrates, such as dextrose, are not strongly "attracted" to the zinc ions so should not pose this problem.[15] The sweetener glycine also appears to be acceptable. Whether other flavorings interfere with the action of zinc remains unknown.

Safety Issues

Zinc seldom causes any immediate side effects other than occasional stomach upset, usually when taken on an empty stomach.

However, make sure that you do not take high doses of zinc for an extended period of time. Long-term use of zinc at dosages of 100 mg or more daily can cause a number of toxic effects, including severe copper deficiency, impaired immunity, heart problems, and anemia.[16–18] The typical 1 to 2 weeks recommended for cold treatment should cause no problems.

If you are taking antibiotics in the quinolone (Cipro or Floxin, for example) or tetracycline family, you should not take zinc within 2 hours before or after your medication dose. Zinc can impair the absorption of those medications.

Other Uses of Zinc

For your information, intriguing evidence suggests that zinc supplements may have other specific benefits beyond killing viruses in your throat. Zinc may reduce symptoms of acne.[19] It seems that people with acne tend to have lower-than-normal levels of zinc in their bodies.[20–23] This fact alone does not prove that taking zinc supplements will help acne, but several small double-blind studies involving a total of over 300 people have found generally positive results.[24–29]

Therapeutic doses of zinc are not recommended for a treatment period longer than 2 weeks.

Zinc may also be helpful in reducing the number, but not the severity, of "sickle-cell crises" in individuals with sickle-cell anemia.[30] With a disease this serious, however, treatment with zinc should not be done except under medical supervision.

Zinc has been tried for rheumatoid arthritis, male fertility, and macular degeneration (a common cause of blindness in the elderly) with mixed results.[31–40] It has been found to speed the healing of stomach ulcers.[41,42]

Other diseases for which there is some evidence (but not yet enough to be meaningful) that zinc works as a treatment include benign prostatic hyperplasia,[43–51] prostatitis,[52] impotence,[53–55] Down's syndrome,[56–58] Alzheimer's disease,[59–62] wound healing,[63–65] inflammatory bowel disease (ulcerative colitis and Crohn's disease),[66–69] tinnitus,[70,71] osteoporosis,[72] diabetes,[73–75] AIDS,[76] anorexia nervosa,[77–80] attention deficit disorder, bladder infection, cataracts, eczema, periodontal disease, and psoriasis.

For more information on using zinc to treat these conditions, see Prima Health's *The Natural Pharmacist: The Natural Health Bible.*

Andrographis: Eastern Medicine Moves West

From the far eastern part of the globe (at least according to European reckoning) comes andrographis, a shrub with a reputation for stimulating the immune system similar to that of echinacea. In fact, it has been referred to as "Indian echinacea." *Andrographis paniculata,* like echinacea, also has a number of other names.[1] In Bengali it is known as *kalmegh;* in Chinese medicine it is called *chaun xin lian,* which translates as "thread-the-heart lotus." Other English names for this plant include *king of bitters* and *chiretta.*

Andrographis grows in plains areas throughout India and other Asian countries. It is most often the above-ground portion of the plant that is used medicinally, although some formulas include extracts of the root.

A Blast from the Past: The Historic Uses of Andrographis

Ayurvedic medicine—one of the oldest medical systems still known in the world today—originated in India and spread throughout neighboring countries. Andrographis has been used for centuries by Ayurvedic physicians to treat infectious diseases such as influenza, malaria, and syphilis. It is also a traditional remedy for a wide variety of problems with the digestive system, including intestinal parasites. Additionally, andrographis appears in a number of Chinese medical formulas, and it is used in traditional Thai herbal medicine as well.[2]

This herb has been used during epidemics, including the Indian flu epidemic of 1919, where andrographis was credited (rightly or wrongly) with saving lives and stopping the spread of the disease.[3]

Ancient Herbal Becomes Modern Medicine

Over the last decade, andrographis has become popular in Scandinavia as a treatment for colds. Most important for our purposes, a few well-designed double-blind studies enrolling a total of about 250 individuals have found that andrographis is indeed effective for this purpose. Although not yet definitive, the evidence we have thus far suggests that, like echinacea, andrographis can improve the symptoms and shorten the duration of colds.

Additionally, one clinical trial found that fairly long-term use of the herb may even help to prevent colds. For more information on using andrographis for cold prevention, see chapter 8.

Clinical Studies

Two double-blind studies have compared andrographis against a placebo, while a third compared it to acetaminophen (most famous as Tylenol).

The first enrolled 50 people with colds and gave them either andrographis or a placebo.[4] It turned out that a full 55% of the treated participants reported that their colds were less intense than usual, while only 19% of those in the placebo group stated this. The treated group averaged only 0.2 days of sick leave, while the untreated patients averaged 1 full day of sick leave. Finally, 75% of the treated patients were well after 5 days, compared to less than 40% in the placebo group. While not stunning, these results are meaningful and indicate that andrographis can indeed function as an effective cold remedy.

Another double-blind placebo-controlled study, this time enrolling 59 people, found similar results.[5] Participants received either 1,200 mg of andrographis (standardized to 4% andrographolides) or a placebo and were evaluated for the severity of cold symptoms such as fatigue, sore muscles, runny nose, headache, and lymph node swelling. By the fourth day of the study, the andrographis group showed significant improvement (compared to the placebo group) in most of the cold symptoms, including sore throat, muscle aches, and fatigue.

Finally, a double-blind study involving 152 adults compared the effectiveness of andrographis (in doses of 3 g per day or 6 g per day, for 7 days) to acetaminophen for sore throat and fever.[6] The higher dose of andrographis decreased symptoms of fever and throat pain about as well as acetaminophen. Interestingly, the lower dose of andrographis (3 g) was not so effective. This kind of dose-related effectiveness is usually considered a strong indication that a treatment really works.

Evidence thus far suggests that andrographis can improve the symptoms and shorten the duration of colds.

A fourth clinical trial also yielded positive results, but this study took quite a different approach, using andrographis not to treat colds, but to prevent altogether their onset in healthy subjects. For more information on some herbs and supplements that might be useful for prevention, see chapter 8.

Although much more research remains to be performed, the results from the clinical trials done with andrographis are quite promising. Hopefully, such research will continue.

How Does Andrographis Work?

As with echinacea, evidence suggests andrographis influences the immune system. In particular, andrographis appears to stimulate both the nonspecific and antigen-specific immune response. This means that it seems to "wake up" two kinds of immune cells: those that attack all invaders indiscriminately, and those that seek out and destroy one particular type of invader they've already identified from a past encounter.

However, as with echinacea, basic research evidence about immune cells doesn't necessarily translate into a meaningful effect. It is not at all certain that andrographis is either an immune strengthener or an immune stimulant. It might have antiviral properties, or work in some other way entirely. We just don't know yet.

What's in Andrographis?

Current evidence suggests that a group of compounds called lactones may be among the active constituents in andrographis. One of these lactones, named andrographolide, is used to standardize the medicines made from the plant. Quite a few laboratory studies have found that andrographolide causes measurable effects in cell cultures and in living creatures. However, because it appears that the whole plant causes a wider range of effects (and more potent effects in some instances) than andrographolides alone, these identified constituents can't be the whole story.[7-9]

Dosage

A typical dose of andrographis is 400 mg 3 times a day. However, doses as high as 1,000 to 2,000 mg have been used in some studies. The andrographis used in most clinical trials was standardized to its content of andrographolide, ranging from 4 to 6%.

Purchasing Andrographis

Andrographis has not yet become so popular that it can be found on every pharmacy shelf. A substantial number of companies offer various formulations for sale on the Internet. As

Andrographis: Coming Soon to a Pharmacy Near You!

It's frustrating to learn about an herb that may well be able to help you get over your cold (or even prevent a cold—see chapter 8 for details) and then learn that it isn't available at the druggist's, or even the local health-food store. Unless you live in Scandinavia or India, it's likely that the only resource you have for andrographis at this time is the Internet. But be of good cheer—this has been the case with a number of other herbs and supplements that are now readily available in most supermarkets. For instance, until the clinical studies that found St. John's wort to be an effective treatment for mild depression were well publicized, local retailers didn't have any reason to stock the product. Now it's everywhere. The same is just beginning to happen with the supplement ipriflavone—it's been popular in some European countries for about a decade but has only recently become available in the United States. Now that the studies on andrographis are beginning to get media attention, you can probably expect to be able to purchase the herb off the pharmacy shelf in the near future.

with most herbal products, some are simply dried plant material, some are extracts; some are standardized, others are not. Oddly enough, those widely advertised standardized products list a much higher content of andrographolide than what was used in the clinical studies—ranging from 10 to 30% (rather than 4 to 6%). This does not necessarily mean that the product is "better." Remember, andrographolide is probably not the only active component in the plant, and we don't know whether increasing the andrographolide content (by substituting it for other unknown but important ingredients) makes the product stronger or weaker.

If you choose to purchase the herb (or anything else, for that matter) via an Internet source, the basic commonsense rules of doing business with unseen, unknown entities apply. It is generally best to do business with companies that list a street address, not just a P.O. box number. If you want to be cautious, perhaps a call to the local Better Business Bureau or Chamber of Commerce where the company is located is in order. As word of andrographis' success in clinical trials becomes more widely known, we may see it becoming more readily available at local stores.

> **Andrographis has not yet become so popular that it can be found on every pharmacy shelf.**

Is Andrographis Safe?

No significant adverse effects have been reported in human studies of andrographis. The 59-person study mentioned in the Clinical Studies section asked participants to report side effects, in addition to monitoring lab tests for liver function, complete blood counts, kidney function, and some other laboratory measures of toxicity. All of their tests came back within normal limits for both the placebo and the andrographis group.[10]

However, full formal safety studies of andrographis have not been completed. For this reason, the herb is not recommended for young children, pregnant or nursing women, or those with severe liver or kidney disease.

Furthermore, animal studies have raised concerns that andrographis may impair fertility. One found that male rats became infertile when fed 20 mg of andrographis powder per day—about 3.5 times the equivalent recommended dose for humans.[11] In this case, the rats stopped producing sperm and exhibited physical changes in some of the testicular cells involved in sperm production. Researchers also detected evidence of degeneration of structures in the testicles. However, another study showed no evidence of testicular toxicity in male rats that were given up to 1 g per kilogram of body weight per day for 60 days—nearly 60 times the usual human dose—so this issue remains unclear.[12]

One group of female mice also did not fare well on andrographis.[13] When fed 2 g per kilogram of body weight daily for 6 weeks (a dose about 120 times higher than the usual human dose), all female mice failed to get pregnant when mated with males of proven fertility. Meanwhile, of the control females, 95.2% got pregnant when mated with a similar group of male mice.

While andrographis is probably not a useful form of birth control, these animal studies warrant further investigation.

Other Uses of Andrographis

Like its Western companion, echinacea, andrographis has traditionally been used for many other complaints (including snakebite!). There has been considerable research into the effectiveness of andrographis for treating other diseases too.

Quite a few studies have evaluated the ability of andrographis to protect the liver against damage caused by such compounds as acetaminophen, alcohol, and carbon tetrachloride[14–21] The findings suggest that andrographis is effective for protecting the liver from these sorts of poisons. In this way, it may be similar to the much more famous liver protective herb milk thistle. In fact, researchers have reported that andrographolide is more potent as a protective agent than silymarin, the active ingredient in milk thistle.

> **Andrographis might be useful for reducing blood pressure, as well as for preventing atherosclerosis.**

Another area where andrographis appears to have potential regards the cardiovascular system. Researchers have found evidence that andrographis might be useful for reducing blood pressure, as well as for preventing atherosclerosis[22–31]

Both traditional uses and some current research suggest andrographis might be useful for the treatment of malaria and certain intestinal parasitic infections[32–34] Investigation into whether it offers potential as an antibiotic has yielded mixed results.[35,36]

Still another area of investigation is into whether or not andrographis might be useful in treating the AIDS virus. Far more research must be done before any conclusions could be reached.

CHAPTER
SIX

Other Herbs and Supplements for Colds: An Alternative Potpourri

S o suppose you've got a stuffy head, aches, and fever, and your determination to loosen this virus' hold on you borders on obsession. You've already read about echinacea, vitamin C, zinc, and andrographis, but you want to try something else. The following treatments are other possible options. Only one, elderberry, has any scientific evidence behind it, and even that is preliminary. Others have the weight of tradition behind them. Do they really work? We don't know yet.

Elderberry: One Small but Encouraging Study

Elderberry *(Sambucus nigra)* is a flowering shrub that produces clusters of creamy-white flowers that mature into dark purple (nearly black) berries somewhat similar in appearance to blueberries, but shiny. It can be found in many areas of North America and Europe.

Historic Uses of Elderberry

Native Americans used tea made from elderberry flowers to treat respiratory infections. They also used the leaves and flowers in poultices applied to wounds, and the bark (suitably aged)

Prove It!

Echinacea is undoubtedly the most thoroughly researched herbal treatment for the common cold. Does this make it better than, for instance, osha root?

Not necessarily. For all we know, osha root may work just as well, or maybe even better. Some people who use osha root swear by it as a remedy for cough and even cold prevention. However, this doesn't prove a thing. The success they have experienced may have had nothing to do with the osha root at all—or may have been a placebo effect, based on their belief that the root would make them well.

Until a number of well-designed, double-blind clinical studies have been done to test it, we just don't know. Choosing between echinacea and one of the less-researched herbs is like deciding whether to keep the $2,000 or take the unseen prize behind door number 3: Until scientific research "opens the door," it's basically gambling.

as a laxative. The berries are frequently made into beverages, pies, and preserves, but they have also been used to treat arthritis.

Elderberry for Colds and Flus

Today, standardized extracts of elderberry are seeing increasing use throughout Europe. Some clinicians feel that elderberry is actually more effective at shortening colds and flus than the far more famous (and better-studied) herb echinacea. According to a preliminary double-blind study performed in Israel, a standardized elderberry extract reduced the recovery time from a particular strain of epidemic influenza by almost half.[1]

Although herbal practitioners usually recommend a tea made from elderberry flowers to treat colds and flus, the extract studied here was produced from the berries.

The researchers who designed this study first investigated cells in petri dishes to determine whether or not the extract could interfere with viral infections. Having found that it could protect cell cultures from damage by viruses, they performed a small clinical trial involving 40 volunteers.

The results were very promising. After only 2 days, 40% of those in the treated group were completely recovered, compared to 16.7% of those who were taking a placebo.

The most obvious drawback to this study is its small size (typical of preliminary studies). Another issue worth noting is that of the 40 initially enrolled for the study, only 27 actually finished, a fact that greatly impairs the credibility of the results from a mathematical point of view. Nonetheless, these early results are definitely impressive enough to warrant larger studies.

How Does Elderberry Work?

The authors of the above study suggest that a chemical in elderberry extract binds to molecules on the surface of viruses, preventing them from attaching to healthy cells. If the virus particles cannot bind to the cells in your body, they cannot enter them, and therefore cannot spread and multiply.

Dosage

The herb used in the clinical study was an extract made from the berry of the elderberry plant, combined with flavorings to make it palatable. This was given at a dose of 4 tablespoons daily for adults, or 2 tablespoons daily for children. Standardized extracts such as this one should be taken according to the directions on the product's label.

Elderberry-flower tea, the more traditional formula for colds and flus, is made by steeping 3 to 5 g of dried flowers in 1 cup of boiling water for 10 to 15 minutes. A typical dosage is 1 cup 3 times daily.

Safety Issues

Elderberries have been used for centuries in cooking. Reported side effects from the flower tea are rare and consist primarily of occasional mild gastrointestinal distress or allergic reactions. Nonetheless, safety in young children, pregnant or nursing women, or those with severe liver or kidney disease is not established.

Other Uses

Elderberry is being studied for potential activity against other viral illnesses as well, including HIV[2] and herpes.[3]

Osha Root: "Colorado Cough Root" and Its Chinese Relatives

Native to high altitudes in the Southwest and Rocky Mountain states, the root of the osha plant (*Ligusticum porteri*) is a traditional Native American remedy for respiratory infections and digestive problems. A related plant, *Ligusticum wallichii,* has a long history of use in Chinese medicine, and most scientific studies on osha were actually performed on this species.

Osha for Colds and Flus

Osha is frequently recommended for use at the first sign of a respiratory infection. Like a sauna, it is said to induce sweating, and according to folk wisdom this may help avert the development of a full-blown cold. Osha is also taken during respiratory infections as a cough suppressant and expectorant, hence the common name "Colorado cough root." Although there have not been any double-blind studies to verify these proposed uses, Chinese research suggests that *Ligusticum wallichii* can relax smooth muscle tissue (perhaps thereby moderating the cough reflex) and inhibit the growth of various bacteria.[4] Whether these findings apply to the *Ligusticum porteri* species as well is unknown.

Osha root is a traditional Native American remedy for respiratory infections and digestive problems.

Dosage

Osha products vary in their concentration and should be taken according to directions on the label. Osha is also available in the form of whole or powdered dried roots, which are steeped in boiling water for 10 to 15 minutes to brew tea, and 1 cup consumed 3 to 4 times daily for cough or congestion.

Safety Issues

Osha is believed to be safe, although the scientific record is sketchy. Traditionally, it is not recommended for use in pregnancy. Safety in young children, nursing women, or those with severe liver or kidney disease has also not been established.

One potential risk with osha is misidentification; the hemlock parsley, a deadly plant with a similar appearance, grows in the same locale. Therefore, don't try to gather this herb yourself.[5]

Other Uses

Like other bitter herbs, osha also tends to improve symptoms of indigestion and increase appetite.

Mullein: A Soothing Beverage, but No Scientific Proof

Also called "grandmother's flannel" for its thick, soft leaves, mullein (*Verbascum thapsus*) is a common wildflower that can grow almost anywhere. It reaches several feet in height and puts up a spike of densely packed tiny yellow flowers. Mullein has served many purposes over the centuries, from making candlewicks to casting out evil spirits, but as medicine it was primarily used to treat diarrhea, respiratory diseases, and hemorrhoids.

Mullein for Colds and Flus

Contemporary herbalists sometimes recommend hot mullein tea for asthma, colds, coughs, and sore throats. Mullein seldom produces dramatic effects, but you'll appreciate its soothing qualities. You can also breathe the steam from a boiling pot of mullein tea. Despite its reputation, not much scientific investigation has focused on this popular herb.

How Does Mullein Work?

Like marshmallow (which we'll discuss later in this chapter), mullein contains a high proportion of mucilage (large sugar molecules that appear to soothe mucous membranes). It also contains saponins that may help loosen mucus.[6]

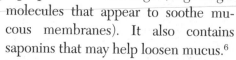

Contemporary herbalists sometimes recommend hot mullein tea for asthma, colds, coughs, and sore throats.

Dosage

To make mullein tea, add 1 to 2 teaspoons of dried leaves and flowers to 1 cup of boiling water and steep for 10 minutes. Make sure to strain the tea before drinking it because fuzzy bits of the herb can stick in your throat and cause an irritating tickle. Mullein is said to be most effective when combined with other herbs of similar qualities, such as yerba santa, marshmallow, cherry bark, and elecampane.

Safety Issues

Mullein leaves and flowers are on the FDA's GRAS (Generally Recognized As Safe) list. Reported side effects are rare. Safety in young children, pregnant or nursing women, or those with severe liver or kidney disease has not been established.

Other Uses

Mullein is also often made into an oily eardrop solution to soothe the pain of ear infections, as long as you're sure the eardrum isn't punctured. But don't expect mullein oil to heal an ear infection: It only relieves the symptoms.

Peppermint: Commission E–Endorsed for Congestion, but No Studies

Peppermint *(Mentha piperita)* is a relative of numerous wild mint plants, deliberately bred in the late 1600s in England to become the delightful tasting plant so well known today. It is widely used as a beverage tea and as a flavoring or scent in a wide variety of products.

Peppermint for Colds and Flus

Peppermint tea has a long history of medicinal use, primarily as a digestive aid, but also for the symptomatic treatment of cough, colds, and fever. Peppermint oil is used for chest congestion—menthol, one of the active ingredients in Vicks VapoRub, is another term for peppermint oil. Germany's Commission E authorizes peppermint oil for, among other uses, relieving mucus congestion of the nose, lungs, and sinuses caused by colds and flus.

Dosage

Peppermint oil, or menthol, is available in several forms for relief of congestion. One is an inhaler stick, which you simply uncap and hold underneath your nose, breathing in the vapors. Another form, which you undoubtedly remember from childhood, is the ointment form (Vicks VapoRub is one brand). This can be rubbed onto your chest or used in a vaporizer.

Safety Issues

Menthol is believed to be safe to inhale, and has been used in this way for many years without any known adverse effects.

Peppermint oil, or menthol, is available in several forms for relief of congestion.

Other Uses

Peppermint oil is also used as a local anesthetic (Solarcaine, Ben-Gay), and, internally, in the treatment of irritable bowel disease, also known as spastic colon. Some evidence suggests that it might be helpful for gallstones.[7] Peppermint is sometimes recommended for the treatment of candida (yeast infections), but there is as yet no real evidence that it works.

Yerba Santa: Strong Folk History, Weak Documentation

Yerba santa *(Eriodictyon californicum)* is a sticky-leafed evergreen that is native to the American Southwest. Spanish priests impressed with its medicinal properties gave the herb its name, which means "holy weed." The aromatic leaves were boiled to make a tea to treat coughs, colds, asthma, pleurisy, tuberculosis, and pneumonia; and a poultice of the leaves was applied to painful joints.

Unlike most medicinal herbs, yerba santa actually has a pleasant taste. It has been used as a general food flavoring and in cough syrups to disguise the bad taste of other ingredients.

Yerba Santa for Colds and Flus

Some modern herbalists regard yerba santa as one of the most effective natural treatments for chronic respiratory problems such as bronchitis and asthma. Unfortunately, no scientific studies of this herb have been reported. About all we can say is that one of its constituents, eriodictyol, appears to be a mild expectorant.[8]

Dosage

Yerba santa tea may be made by adding 1 teaspoon of crushed leaves to a cup of boiling water and steeping for half an hour. Drink 3 cups a day until symptoms subside. Because many of its resinous constituents do not dissolve in water, however, alcoholic tinctures of yerba santa may be more effective. Such tinctures should be taken according to the directions on the label.

Safety Issues

Yerba santa is on the FDA's GRAS list for use as a food flavoring. There have been no reports of significant side effects or adverse reactions,[9] except for the inevitable occasional allergic reaction. Nonetheless, the herb's safety for young children, pregnant or nursing women, or those with severe liver or kidney disease has not been established.

Unlike most medicinal herbs, yerba santa actually has a pleasant taste.

Other Uses

Yerba santa is occasionally used topically as a treatment for poison ivy.[10]

Marshmallow: A Sore Throat Soother

The similarity in name between the herb marshmallow (*Althaea officinalis*) and the sweet treat is more than a coincidence, although the modern sugar puffball no longer bears much similarity in taste and appearance to the old-fashioned candy flavored with marshmallow herb.

Besides inspiring makers of campfire food, the marshmallow has also been used medicinally since ancient Greece. Hippocrates spoke of it as a treatment for bruises and blood loss, and subsequent Roman physicians recommended marshmallow for toothaches, insect bites, chilblains, and irritated skin. In medieval Europe, herbalists used marshmallow to soothe toothaches, coughs, sore throats, chapped skin, indigestion, and diarrhea.

Marshmallow for Colds and Flus

Modern herbalists often recommend marshmallow for respiratory problems, such as coughs, colds, and asthma. Like mullein, the herb contains very high levels of large sugar molecules called mucilage, which appear to exert a soothing effect on mucous membranes. While marshmallow is more a symptomatic treatment than a cure, its ability to soothe a raw throat can be very welcome. No double-blind studies have been reported at this time.

Dosage

Marshmallow can be made into a soothing tea by steeping roots overnight in water and diluting to taste. This tea can be drunk as desired for symptomatic relief. Alternatively, you can take marshmallow in capsules (5 to 6 g daily) or in tincture, according to label directions.

> **Modern herbalists often recommend marshmallow for respiratory problems, such as coughs, colds, and asthma.**

Safety Issues

Marshmallow is believed to be entirely safe. It is approved for use in foods, and its chemical makeup does not suggest any but benign effects.[11] However, detailed safety studies have not been performed. One study suggests that marshmallow might slightly lower blood sugar levels.[12] For this reason, people with diabetes should use caution when taking marshmallow. Safety in young children, pregnant or nursing women, or those with severe liver or kidney disease has not been established.

Other Uses

Marshmallow is also recommended for digestive problems, and sometimes as an ointment for ulcers to reduce discomfort.

Kudzu

Kudzu (*Pueraria lobata*) has become an invasive pest in the United States; in China, it is used as both food and medicine.

One classic Chinese herbal formula containing kudzu is recommended for the treatment of colds accompanied by pain in the neck. It is obtainable either through a practitioner of Chinese herbal medicine (the preferable source), or over the counter in some stores.

Kudzu, an invasive pest in the United States, is used as both food and medicine in China.

Based on its extensive food use, kudzu is believed to be reasonably safe. However, safety in young children, pregnant or nursing women, or those with severe kidney or liver disease has not been established.

Ginger

Chinese herbalists have used ginger *(Zingiber officinale)* to treat a variety of respiratory conditions, including coughs and the early stages of colds. Traditional Chinese herbalists believe hot ginger tea taken at the first sign of a cold offers the possibility of averting the infection, but there is as yet no scientific documentation for this idea. Ginger is on the FDA's GRAS list as a food, and the treatment dosages of ginger are comparable to dietary usages.

Slippery Elm

Like marshmallow and mullein, slippery elm *(Ulmus rubra, Ulmus fulva)* was used as a treatment for sore throat, coughs, and dryness of the lungs. It's primarily used today as a cough lozenge, widely available in pharmacies. Other than occasional allergic reactions, slippery elm has not been associated with any toxicity. However, its safety has never been formally studied. Safety in young children, pregnant or nursing women, or those with severe liver or kidney disease has not been established.

Yarrow

Yarrow (*Achillea millefolium*) has also been used traditionally as treatment for respiratory infections. Like osha, yarrow tea is commonly taken at the first sign of a cold or flu to bring on sweating and, according to tradition, to ward off infection.

To make yarrow tea, steep 1 to 2 teaspoons of dried herb per cup of water. Combination products should be taken according to label instructions.

No clear toxicity has been associated with yarrow.[13] The FDA has expressed concern about a toxic constituent of yarrow known as thujone and permits only thujone-free yarrow extracts for use in beverages. Nonetheless, the common spice sage contains more thujone than yarrow, and the FDA lists sage as generally recognized as safe.

There are no reports of serious side effects with yarrow. Safety in young children, pregnant or nursing women, or those with severe liver or kidney disease has not been established.

Garlic

Garlic (*Allium sativum*) has a traditional reputation for preventing colds and warding off vampires. Neither use (especially not the vampire one) is yet supported by any reliable evidence.

One report stated that garlic can improve some aspects of immune system activity, including white blood cell count, natural killer cell activity, and phagocytosis, much like what was described for echinacea.[14] However, this evidence does not really establish that eating garlic will improve immunity.

Garlic has been found to work as a topical antibiotic, meaning that it kills bacteria when it touches them (like Bacitracin, bleach, and iodine). It does not appear, however, that garlic works like penicillin as a whole-body antibiotic when you eat it. Furthermore, since colds are generally caused by viruses, not by bacteria, it really wouldn't matter in terms of cold treatment.

Of course, there have always been those who believe garlic prevents colds simply because it keeps contagious coworkers from hanging around and infecting you!

Because garlic is widely consumed as a food, it is generally believed to be safe. However, garlic decreases blood clotting, and you should not combine it with blood-thinning drugs such as Coumadin (warfarin), heparin, or perhaps even aspirin. It is also possible that garlic could cause bleeding problems if combined with natural blood thinners, such as ginkgo and high-dose vitamin E. Excessive garlic intake can also cause stomach distress, nervousness, gas, and bloating.

Goldenseal: A Misrepresented Herb

Goldenseal falls into a category all to itself here: It is widely sold in combination with echinacea as a treatment for colds, but for this purpose it has neither scientific evidence nor a traditional history of usage.

The origin of this incorrect formulation appears to have gone as follows: Antibiotics are useful for colds (wrong), goldenseal is an antibiotic (partially wrong), and therefore goldenseal is good for colds. Actually, like garlic, goldenseal is only a topical antibiotic, used traditionally for skin wounds. In any case, colds are caused by viruses, which don't respond to antibiotics.

An alternative explanation sometimes given for using goldenseal claims that the herb can strengthen the immune system. However, there is no evidence that this is so, and it doesn't accord with the traditional uses of the herb.

It is true that goldenseal was traditionally believed to have a healing effect on mucous membranes. For this reason, an old-fashioned herbalist might have recommended it in the later stages of a cold, but not for use at the beginning.

Since goldenseal is currently an endangered plant, you should avoid using it for colds and flus; it really isn't appropriate and you may contribute to the loss of this plant species.

Another characteristic incorrectly assigned to goldenseal is that it can block a positive drug test. This mistaken belief has led to enormous sales of the herb, and probably to numerous problems with the law, since it doesn't work.

Adaptogens for
Colds and Flus:
Potential for Prevention

Most of the treatments covered in previous sections are intended to help get rid of your cold a little sooner or to make your sore throat not so sore and your stuffy nose not so stuffy. But let's face it—no one wants to get sick in the first place. What can you do to just avoid the illness altogether? This chapter and the next one have a few ideas for you along those lines.

As you may recall from chapter 1, the term "adaptogen" describes a hypothetical treatment that should help the body adapt to stresses of various kinds—whether heat, cold, exertion, trauma, sleep deprivation, toxic exposure, radiation, infection, or psychological stress. Furthermore, an adaptogen should cause no side effects, be effective in treating a wide variety of illnesses, and help return an organism toward balance no matter what may have gone wrong.

Perhaps the only factor that actually has this effect is a healthy lifestyle: eating right, exercising regularly, and generally living a life of balance and moderation. However, some people feel certain that ginseng is an adaptogen, capable of producing similarly universal benefits.

In addition, some consider a number of other herbs, including astragalus, ashwagandha, and maitake, to be adaptogens as well.

Ginseng

There are actually three different herbs commonly called ginseng: Asian or Korean ginseng *(Panax ginseng),* American ginseng *(Panax quinquefolius),* and Siberian "ginseng" *(Eleutherococcus senticosus).* The latter herb is actually not ginseng at all, but the Russian scientists responsible for promoting it believe that it functions identically.

Asian ginseng is a perennial herb with a taproot resembling the human body (see figure 3). It grows in northern China, Korea, and Russia; its close relative, *Panax quinquefolius,* is cultivated in the United States. Because ginseng must be grown for 5 years before it is harvested, it commands a high price, with top-quality roots easily selling for more than $10,000. Dried, unprocessed ginseng root is called "white ginseng," and steamed, heat-dried root is "red ginseng." Chinese herbalists believe that each form has its own particular benefits.

At least one well-designed study suggests regular use of ginseng might help prevent colds and flus.

Ginseng is widely regarded by the public as a stimulant; but according to most serious users of the herb, that isn't an apt description. In traditional Chinese herbology, *Panax ginseng* was used to strengthen the digestion and the lungs, calm the spirit, and increase overall energy. When the Russian scientist Israel I. Brekhman became interested in the herb prior to World War II, he came up with a new idea about ginseng. He decided it was an adaptogen.

Interestingly, traditional Chinese medicine (where ginseng was first used) does not entirely support this idea. There is no

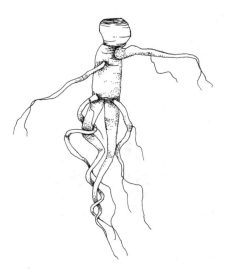

Figure 3. *Asian ginseng root* (Panax ginseng)

one-size-fits-all in Chinese medical theory. Like any other herb, ginseng is said to be helpful for those people who need its particular effects, and neutral or harmful for others. But in Europe, Brekhman's concept has taken hold, and ginseng is widely believed to be a universal adaptogen.

In the 1940s, Brekhman decided that a much less expensive herb, *Eleutherococcus senticosus,* is just as good as ginseng. A thorny bush that grows much more rapidly than true ginseng, this later received the misleading name of "Siberian" or "Russian ginseng." Contrary to some reports, its chemical makeup is completely unrelated to that of *Panax ginseng.*

Prevention of Colds and Flus with Ginseng

According to at least one well-designed study, regular use of ginseng might help prevent colds and flus. In this double-blind placebo-controlled trial, researchers examined whether a standardized extract of ginseng root would improve immune responses to a flu vaccine.[1] The trial enrolled 227 participants at three medical offices in Milan, Italy. Half were given ginseng at

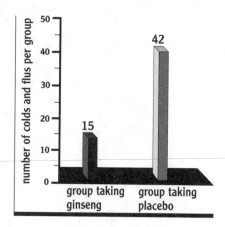

Figure 4. *Double-blind study shows that ginseng reduced the number of colds and flus (Scaglione et al., 1996)*

a dosage of 100 mg daily, the other half a placebo. Four weeks into the study, all participants received influenza vaccine.

After the vaccine, the placebo group reported 42 cases of colds or flus, but the treated group reported only 15 cases of colds or flus, a difference that was statistically significant (see figure 4). In addition, the treated group had a significantly greater rise in antibodies that fight influenza.

Researchers noted a few minor adverse effects during the study, the most prominent of which was insomnia. They also followed 24 laboratory-measured "safety parameters" and noted no significant difference between the two groups for these. Their conclusion was that ginseng improved immune response while having minimal adverse effects.

Older scientific studies have also found that ginseng can prevent colds, but these studies were not designed properly. Even though some of the clinical studies included enormous numbers of participants, most were not double-blind or even controlled, which makes the results nearly meaningless.

For example, one widely quoted study followed over 50,000 employees at a Soviet automobile plant who were given

Eleutherococcus (which, as mentioned on page 75, isn't true ginseng) daily during November and December. Plant records showed that the frequency of respiratory infections fell by 40%.[2] However, without a control group, it isn't clear how many infections would have been expected without any treatment. Perhaps it was a milder winter, for example. Furthermore, since the participants knew they were being treated, the placebo effect was given full reign. If the subjects had been given dried shoe leather described as a healing herb, they would have undoubtedly reported fewer illnesses. The scientists reporting the results would likely be similarly biased.

It doesn't matter how many people were involved: Without a control group and double-blind design, both the participants and the researchers are subject to the power of suggestion. No such study can prove much.

Still more of the studies done on ginseng used animals. While animal studies can be very useful, in most of these studies ginseng was injected directly into the abdomen.[3] This doesn't really give us an accurate idea of how it will work when we take it by mouth. It not only enters the body without going through the digestive tract, but for all we know, an injection into the abdomen may itself stimulate numerous bodily changes.

Taken in its entirety, the scientific record on ginseng is intriguing but not conclusive. If some of the money spent on animal and non-double-blind human studies had been used to fund more double-blind studies in humans, we might know a lot more.

How Does Ginseng Work?

Evidence suggests that ginseng may be able to increase the activity of the immune system. A number of the studies using cell cultures, animals, and human volunteers have found that ginseng extract increases the production of several types of immune cells and also increases phagocytosis (the "swallowing" of foreign bodies by specialized immune cells).[4] Increased phagocytosis and numbers of immune cells may not necessarily translate into a real improvement in immunity—for instance, it doesn't seem to work that way with echinacea. However, the clinical study discussed above found that ginseng did seem to improve resistance to disease. The increase in immune system response is one theory researchers offer to explain how ginseng is raising our resistance to illness, but more research will be needed before anyone can state with certainty that this is really the way it happens.

Dosage

The typical recommended daily dosage of *Panax ginseng* is 1 to 2 g of raw herb, or 200 mg daily of an extract standardized to contain 4 to 7% ginsenosides. Some herbalists recommend taking periodic "breaks" from ginseng, but the recommended duration of these breaks and length of time between them seems to be a matter of widely varied opinion. No studies support the need for taking ginseng in this off-and-on way.

Most of the studies of ginseng used products containing standardized ginseng extracts. Although we don't know how to tell if one form of ginseng is more effective than another based on this standardization, such extracts do ensure that you're buying the plant you think you are buying and not paying a premium price for Asian ginseng but getting the less expensive *Eleutherococcus*. (This, of course, assumes that the manufacturer honestly reports the results of standardized testing, which is not required by U.S. regulatory authorities.)

The dose for *Eleutherococcus* is 300 to 400 mg per day of standardized solid extract (standardized on eleutherosides B and E), or 4 to 5 ml of tincture twice per day. If you are taking a dried, nonstandardized product (powdered root or rhizome), take 2 to 3 g per day.

Finally, because *Panax ginseng* is so expensive, some products actually contain very little of the herb. Adulteration with other herbs and even caffeine is not unusual.[5]

Safety Issues

The various forms of ginseng appear to be nontoxic, both in the short and the long term, according to the results of studies in

---

Potential Interactions with Ginseng

Talk to your physician or pharmacist about using ginseng if you are taking any of the following conventional drugs:

- **Drugs processed by an enzyme called "CYP 3A4":** Ask your physician or pharmacist whether you are taking any medications of this type since ginseng might interfere with them.
- **Insulin:** Taking ginseng may require you to reduce your insulin dosage.
- **Digoxin:** *Eleutherococcus* may interfere with blood tests for digoxin levels.
- **Coumadin (warfarin):** Ginseng might decrease its effect.
- **MAO inhibitor drugs:** It is possible that a ginseng product might cause hypertension if combined with these drugs, especially if it is contaminated with caffeine.

---

mice, rats, chickens, and dwarf pigs. Ginseng also does not seem to be carcinogenic.[6–8]

Reported side effects are rare. The double-blind Italian study found few side effects other than occasional insomnia.[9]

There have been reports of menstrual abnormalities and/or breast tenderness in some women taking Asian ginseng.[10,11]

Unconfirmed reports suggest that very high doses of ginseng (greater than 10 times the normal dose) can raise blood pressure, increase heart rate, and possibly cause other significant effects. Whether some of these cases were actually caused by caffeine mixed in with ginseng remains unclear, but we do know that some manufacturers have at times added caffeine to their ginseng products (and "forgotten" to put it on the labels). Ginseng allergy can also occur, as can allergy to any other substance. Although allergic reactions would be extremely uncommon, highly allergic individuals should introduce ginseng into their lives cautiously just in case.

In 1979, an article was published in the *Journal of the American Medical Association* claiming that people can become addicted to ginseng and develop blood pressure elevation, nervousness, sleeplessness, diarrhea, and hypersexuality.[12] This report has since been thoroughly discredited and shouldn't be taken seriously.[13,14]

Some evidence suggests that ginseng can interfere with drug metabolism (see the sidebar, page 79), specifically drugs processed by an enzyme called "CYP 3A4."[15] Ask your physician or pharmacist whether you are taking any medications of this type. There have been specific reports of ginseng interacting with MAO inhibitor drugs as well,[16] although it is not clear whether it was the ginseng or a contaminant that caused the problem. There has also been one report of ginseng reducing the anticoagulant effects of Coumadin (warfarin).[17] Additionally, there has been a report of *Eleutherococcus* interfering with a test for blood levels of digoxin, a drug used to regulate heart rhythm and treat congestive heart failure.[18]

Safety in young children, pregnant or nursing women, or those with severe liver or kidney disease has not been established. Interestingly, Chinese tradition suggests that ginseng should not be used by pregnant or nursing mothers, and Russian tradition suggests that ginseng should not be used by those under 40.

Other Uses

Ginseng has also been investigated for treatment of diabetes, improving mental function and sports performance, and prevention of cancer. A double-blind clinical study evaluated the effects of *Panax ginseng* (at dosages of 100 mg or 200 mg daily) on 36 people with adult-onset diabetes.[19] The results showed increased physical activity that translated into improvements in blood sugar control.

The results of a double-blind placebo-controlled clinical study on ginseng's effect on mental function found that ginseng improved abstract thinking ability but did not affect reaction time, memory, concentration, or overall subjective experience.[20] Neither *Panax ginseng* nor an *Eleutherococcus* formulation produced improvement in physical performance when tested for the purpose.[21,22]

A recent study on ginseng and cancer prevention has been widely publicized, but a close look at the data arouses some suspicions. This study was performed in South Korea and followed a total of 4,587 men and women aged 39 years and older from 1987 to 1991.[23] People who regularly consumed *Panax ginseng* were compared with otherwise similar individuals (matched in sex, age, alcohol use, smoking, and education and economic status) who did not.

Ginseng has been investigated for treating diabetes, improving mental function and sports performance, and preventing cancer.

The results were impressive—maybe a little too impressive. Those who used ginseng showed a 60% decrease in risk of death from cancer. Lung cancer and gastric cancer were particularly reduced. The more ginseng consumed, the greater the effect. However, use of ginseng fewer than 3 times per year caused a 54% reduction in cancer risk! It seems difficult to believe that so occasional a use of ginseng could reduce cancer mortality by more than half. A controlled study is needed to confirm, or refute, this study's findings.

Astragalus

Dried and sliced thin, the root of the astragalus plant *(Astragalus membranaceus)* is a common component of traditional Chinese herbal formulas. According to Chinese medical theory, astragalus "strengthens the spleen, blood and Qi, raises the yang Qi of the spleen and stomach, and stabilizes the exterior."[24] Don't worry if you didn't understand what you just read. No one without training in the unique Chinese approach to illness would! The belief that astragalus can strengthen immunity has its basis in the "stabilize the exterior" part, which means helping to create a defensive shield against infection.

Preventing Colds and Flus with Astragalus

In the United States, astragalus has been presented as an immune stimulant useful for treating colds and flus. Many people have come to believe that they should take astragalus, like echinacea, at the first sign of a cold.

However, there is no real scientific basis for using astragalus for this purpose. Furthermore, according to Chinese healing tradition, astragalus formulas should not be taken during the early stage of infections. To do so is said to resemble "locking the chicken coop with the fox inside," causing the infection to be "driven deeper." Rather, astragalus is supposedly only appropriate for use while you're healthy, for the purpose of preventing future illnesses. Since it was Chinese usage that led to the recognition of astragalus as a medicinal herb, perhaps these traditions should be taken seriously. Although tradition suggests that astragalus should always be used in combination with other herbs, modern Chinese investigators have found various intriguing effects when astragalus is taken by itself. Extracts of astragalus have been shown to stimulate parts of the immune system in mice and humans, and to increase the survival time of mice infected with various diseases.[25,26] But none of this constitutes evidence that astragalus can prevent colds.

Traditional Chinese medicine warns against using astragalus in cases of acute infections.

Dosage

The traditional method of using astragalus involves boiling 9 to 30 g per day of dried root to make tea. Newer products use an alcohol-and-water extraction method to produce an extract standardized to astragaloside content, but researchers and health practitioners haven't yet agreed on the proper percentage.

Safety Issues

Astragalus appears to be relatively nontoxic. High one-time doses, as well as long-term administration, have not caused significant harmful effects.[27] Side effects are rare and generally limited to the usual mild gastrointestinal distress or allergic reactions.

As mentioned on page 82, traditional Chinese medicine warns against using astragalus in cases of acute infections. Other traditional contraindications include "deficient yin patterns with heat signs" and "exterior excess heat patterns." Since these warnings don't mean much to anyone without an extensive education in Chinese medicine, we recommend using astragalus only under the supervision of a qualified Chinese herbalist.

Safety in young children, pregnant or nursing women, or those with severe liver or kidney disease is not established.

Other Uses

Preliminary research suggests that astragalus might also be useful in treating atherosclerosis, hyperthyroidism, hypertension, insomnia, diabetes, chronic active hepatitis, genital herpes, AIDS, and the side effects of cancer chemotherapy.[28–33] However, none of these suggestions can be regarded as proven.

Ashwagandha

Ashwagandha *(Withania somniferum)* is sometimes called "Indian ginseng," not because it's related botanically (it's closer to potatoes and tomatoes), but because its uses are similar. Like ginseng, ashwagandha is a "tonic herb" traditionally believed capable of generally strengthening the body. However, it is believed to be milder and less stimulating than ginseng.

Preventing Colds and Flus with Ashwagandha

Like ginseng, ashwagandha is said to increase the body's resistance to infection when it is taken for an extended period of time. Clinicians who use ashwagandha often report that it is as effective as ginseng, but gentler in action. However, we have almost no scientific evidence to which we can turn.

Ashwagandha is a "tonic herb" traditionally believed capable of generally strengthening the body.

Researchers in one study fed ashwagandha to mice with aspergilliosis infections.[34] Mice that were given the herb survived longer than mice that did not receive it. The researchers believed these results were due to improvements in some aspects of immune system activity, including phagocytosis.

Dosage

A typical dosage of ashwagandha is 1 teaspoon of powder twice a day, boiled in milk or water. Herbalists often recommend that those who are young or especially weak should take a lower dosage.

Safety Issues

Although formal scientific safety studies have not been completed, ashwagandha appears to be safe when taken in normal doses. However, because some of the constituents of ashwagandha can make you drowsy, it should not be combined with sedative drugs. The herb may also have some steroid-like activity at high dosages.[35] Safety in young children, pregnant or nursing women, or those with severe liver or kidney disease is not yet established.

Other Uses

Highly preliminary studies suggest that ashwagandha may reduce the negative effects of stress, inhibit inflammation, lower

cholesterol, increase sexual performance, produce mild seda-
tion (a benefit useful for those troubled by insomnia or anxiety),
increase hemoglobin levels, and inhibit tumor growth.[36–39] Further studies remain to be performed to evaluate these potential
benefits. Ashwagandha has also been suggested as a treatment
for infertility.

Maitake

Maitake *(Grifola frondosa)* is a medicinal mushroom used in
Japan as a general promoter of robust health. Like the reishi
fungus (which we'll discuss next), innumerable healing powers
have been attributed to maitake, ranging from curing cancer to
preventing heart disease. Unfortunately, there hasn't been
enough reliable research yet to determine whether any of these
ancient beliefs are really true. Traditionally, maitake was used
as a tonic to promote wellness and energy, to fight infections,
and to adapt to stress. On this basis, some modern herbalists
have decided that maitake must be an adaptogen.

Preventing Colds and Flus with Maitake

As for most of the other alleged adaptogens, we lack definitive
scientific evidence to show us that maitake really raises our immunity to colds, flus, or other illnesses. Those studies that have
been done have been laboratory
research, not clinical trials. Most investigation has focused on the polysaccharide constituents of maitake. This
family of substances is known to affect
the human immune system in complex
ways. It has been suggested that
maitake's polysaccharides may stimulate immune system activity, but we
are not sure that this is true. At this
time, we have no definitive studies.

**Maitake is a medi-
cinal mushroom
used in Japan as a
general promoter
of robust health.**

Still, without waiting for evidence, many practitioners recommend maitake as an immune system stimulant.

Dosage

Maitake is an edible mushroom that can be eaten as food or made into tea. A typical dosage of dried maitake in capsule or tablet form is 3 to 7 g daily.

Safety Issues

Maitake is widely believed to be safe, although formal safety studies have not been performed. Safety in young children, pregnant or nursing women, or those with severe liver or kidney disease has not been established.

Other Uses

Of the polysaccharides found in maitake, one in particular, beta-D-glucan, has been studied for its potential benefit in treating cancer and AIDS.[40,41] Highly preliminary studies also suggest that maitake may be useful in treating diabetes, hypertension (high blood pressure), and high cholesterol. However, no real evidence as yet tells us that maitake is effective for these or any other illnesses.

Reishi

The tree fungus known as reishi (*Ganoderma lucidum*) has a long history of use in China and Japan as a semi-magical healing herb. Many stories tell of people with severe illnesses journeying immense distances to find reishi, which is more revered than ginseng and, until recently, more rare. Presently, reishi is artificially cultivated and widely available in stores that sell herb products.

Preventing Colds and Flus with Reishi

Contemporary herbalists regard reishi as capable of helping the body to resist stress of all kinds—in other words, as an adaptogen. As such, it is believed to strengthen immunity against infection. However, while a great deal of basic scientific research has explored the chemical constituents of reishi, reliable double-blind studies are lacking. Whether or not reishi will keep away a cold or influenza hasn't yet been determined.

Dosage

The usual dosage of reishi is 2 to 6 g per day of raw fungus, or if you're taking a concentrated extract, you should follow the manufacturer's recommendations. Reishi should be taken with meals. It is often combined with related fungi, such as shiitake, hoelen, or polyporus. Some people take reishi continually for its presumed overall health benefits; these benefits are said to develop only after about 1 to 2 weeks of regular use.

Contemporary herbalists regard reishi as capable of helping the body resist stress of all kinds.

Safety Issues

Reishi appears to be extremely safe. Occasional side effects include mild digestive upset, dry mouth, and skin rash. Reishi can "thin" the blood slightly, and therefore should not be combined with drugs such as Coumadin (warfarin) or heparin. Safety in young children, pregnant or nursing women, or those with severe liver or kidney disease has not been established.

Other Uses

Reishi is marketed as a cure-all, said to prevent and treat cancer, restore normal immune function in autoimmune diseases (such as *myasthenia gravis),* improve symptoms of asthma and bronchitis, overcome viral hepatitis, prevent and treat cardiovascular disease, improve mental function, heal ulcers, and prevent altitude sickness. However, no real evidence demonstrates that reishi is effective for any of these conditions.

Suma

Suma *(Pfaffia paniculata)* is a large ground vine native to Central and South America. Native peoples have long used suma, sometimes called "Brazilian ginseng," in the belief that it promotes robust health and can treat practically all illnesses. They called it *Para Toda,* which means "for all things."[42]

Preventing Colds and Flus with Suma

Suma's ancient reputation has generated worldwide interest. However, little formal scientific investigation has been performed at this time. According to many contemporary herbalists, suma helps one adapt to stress and fight infection, so it is sometimes used to treat people with a low resistance to illness.

Dosage

A typical dosage of suma is 500 mg twice daily. It is usually taken for an extended period of time.

Safety Issues

Suma has not been associated with any serious adverse reactions. However, comprehensive safety studies have not been undertaken. Safety in young children, pregnant or nursing women, or those with severe liver or kidney disease has not been established.

Other Uses

Along with other adaptogens, Russian Olympic athletes have used suma with the belief that it will enhance sports performance. In the United States, suma is often recommended as a general strengthener of the body, as well as for the treatment of chronic fatigue syndrome, menopausal symptoms, ulcers, anxiety, and menstrual problems. The herb also enjoys a considerable reputation as an aphrodisiac. None of these ideas has been clinically tested.

Preventing Colds and Flus with Echinacea?

Echinacea has been widely used to prevent colds and flus. You may know someone who takes it throughout the cold season, and swears by the results. However, the evidence from scientific studies is contradictory at best. Three published double-blind studies of the herb's ability to prevent illness do not offer any real evidence that it works. Furthermore, an as-yet-unpublished study done at Bastyr College in Washington actually found a 20% higher incidence of colds and flus in the group taking echinacea compared to those on a placebo.

The most recent of the three published studies was a double-blind placebo-controlled trial involving 302 healthy volunteers.[43] Each participant was given an alcohol tincture containing either *E. purpurea* root, *E. angustifolia* root, or a placebo for a period of 12 weeks. The results showed that *E. purpurea* was associated with perhaps a 20% decrease in the number of

Native peoples have long used suma, believing that it promotes robust health and can treat practically all illnesses.

people who got sick, and *E. angustifolia* with a 10% decrease. However, the difference between the treatment groups and those receiving the placebo was not statistically significant. The problem is that the comparative benefit, if any, was so small that it could have been due to chance alone.

In another double-blind study, a similarly slight benefit was seen among participants already especially likely to catch cold.[44] In the study group as a whole, a mixture containing *E. angustifolia* did not significantly decrease the number of colds. However, of the total 609 people studied, 363 were rated as particularly infection-prone, based on the number of infections each had developed the winter before. This relatively high-risk group *did* show a statistically significant reduction in the total number of colds when compared with the control group. The change, while not gigantic, was significant: The infection-prone students developed on average 20% fewer colds. (You might ask why a 20% improvement is significant in this study, while it was found not significant in the previous study. The explanation involves the number of people enrolled in the trial. The more people involved in a study, the more you trust relatively slight observed benefits.)

An earlier double-blind placebo-controlled study also attempted to discover whether echinacea can prevent infections from starting.[45] This 8-week study included 108 people, 54 of whom took *E. purpurea* and 54 of whom did not. Those in the treated group overall experienced a longer period of health before the first cold—40 versus 25 days. Unfortunately, while this study is widely quoted as clear evidence that echinacea is effective, from a mathematical point of view, the apparent benefit was again not statistically significant.

Take echinacea when you get sick to help you get better faster, but don't expect it to prevent colds.

To make matters worse, an as-yet-unpublished study of 200 people, intended to evaluate echinacea's preventive action, found an actual 20% higher incidence of flus and colds among the population taking echinacea as compared with the placebo group![46]

What can we make of a body of research where some studies report a mostly insignificant 10% to 20% reduction in colds, but another finds a 20% increase in colds? Here's the most likely explanation: If echinacea works at all for prevention, it doesn't work very well. Take echinacea when you get sick to help you get better faster, but don't expect it to prevent colds.

Vitamins, Minerals, and Andrographis for Prevention

S ince you are still reading this book, you must *really* hate getting sick! Here are a few further treatments you can use to "germ-proof" your immune system.

Andrographis, vitamin E, zinc, and vitamin C have all been studied to see whether they could keep colds or flus from ever getting started. All these treatments have been found to help chase such illness away once it has developed, as you read in chapters 3, 4, and 5. So why not use them to ward off sickness in the first place? After all, if you find that a large, trained gorilla is good at evicting unwanted houseguests, it stands to reason that having the gorilla there all the time might prevent guests from coming to visit in the first place. And in some cases, it seems to be true.

Andrographis: Reduced Numbers of Colds with a Low-Dose Extract

For a complete description of *Andrographis paniculata,* a medicinal herb from India, and its use in treating colds, see chapter 5. Now we will discuss a study of the use of andrographis for prevention.

Preventing Colds with Andrographis

According to one double-blind placebo-controlled study, andrographis may increase resistance to colds.[1] A total of 107 students, all age 18, participated in this 3-month-long trial using a dried extract of andrographis. Fifty-four of the participants took two 100 mg tablets standardized to 5.6% andrographolide daily—considerably less than the 1,200 to 6,000 mg per day that has been used in studies on treatment of colds. The other 53 students were given placebo tablets with a coating identical to the treatment. Then, once a week throughout the study, a clinician evaluated all the participants for cold symptoms.

For the first 2 months of the study, the difference between the two groups was not significant from a statistical point of view. However, during each month the students taking the andrographis showed fewer respiratory illnesses than did those on a placebo. By the end of the trial, only 16 people in the group using andrographis had experienced colds, compared to 33 of the placebo group participants. This difference was statistically significant, amounting to a 33% reduction in occurrence of colds with use of the andrographis.

With these encouraging results, further study of andrographis as a preventative for colds seems well worth pursuing. Researchers still have many questions to answer in this regard. For example, during the first month of this study, the treatment group had 8% fewer colds than did the placebo group. That difference increased to 23% by the second month; and by the third, the andrographis users experienced 33% fewer colds. If the study had continued for 6 months, or even longer, would the difference be even greater? Would a study involving more participants show the differences more clearly? And would a dose larger than the 200 mg given be even more effective in preventing colds?

How Does Andrographis Work for Prevention?

Andrographis has been found to stimulate immune cells, both the type that "remember" previous attackers and the type that respond more generally to any invader. This increase in immune response may be responsible for andrographis's apparent protective effect—but we're waiting for more studies to fill the gaps in what we know before we can say for sure.

Dosage and Safety Issues

The dosage used in the study mentioned above—200 mg daily, standardized to 5.6% andrographolide—appeared to be effective, yet this is a dose lower than that suggested for treating colds. Whether this is the best dose for cold prevention is not known; further studies are needed to determine this.

None of the participants dropped out of the study during the 3-month trial, which suggests that none experienced noticeable side effects; the authors, however, did not report on side effects.

Complete information on dosage and safety issues for this herb can be found in chapter 5.

Vitamin E: More Antibodies, Fewer Infections

The best food sources of vitamin E are polyunsaturated vegetable oils, seeds, nuts, and whole grains. Vitamin E is actually a family of compounds called *tocopherols.* It's a fairly big family, with a lot of little tocopherols—but the most common form used in supplements is a synthetic form called *DL-alpha tocopherol.* Some people feel that natural vitamin E is better for you, but as yet we have no proof of this (see the sidebar, page 94). To get a therapeutic dosage of vitamin E you need to take a supplement; you really can't get enough in food to produce this potential benefit.

To get a therapeutic dosage of vitamin E, you need to take a supplement.

Increasing Immunity with Vitamin E

A recent double-blind study suggests that vitamin E may beef up your body's defenses against disease. This study involved 88

Is Natural Vitamin E Better Than Synthetic?

Some evidence suggests that natural forms of vitamin E are more effective than the man-made DL-alpha-tocopherol.[2–4] Natural vitamin E comes from foods we eat, and contains beta-, delta-, and gamma-tocopherols, as well as other compounds in the tocopherol family (think of them as cousins), such as tocotrienols. Natural vitamin E also differs from the synthetic kind in another way as well. Organic chemicals can come in two forms, like left and right gloves. These are called D- (for *dextro,* or right-handed) and L- (for *levo,* or left-handed) isomers. Natural vitamin E is all the D form. Synthetic vitamin E contains a mixture of D- and L-forms.

Researchers have suggested that the best vitamin E supplement would be a natural mixture of tocopherols including alpha-, delta-, and gamma- ("mixed tocopherols"), all of which should be in the D form. However, all the scientific evidence we have for the effectiveness of vitamin E supplements comes from studies using synthetic DL-alpha-tocopherol, so at this point we have no direct confirmation that natural vitamin E is better.

adults over age 65, all of whom were considered to be healthy and have normally functioning immune systems. The subjects were given either a placebo or vitamin E at 60 IU, 200 IU, or 800 IU daily.[5] (By comparison, the dietary requirements for vitamin E range from about 10 to 15 IU daily.) The researchers then gave all participants immunizations against hepatitis B, tetanus, diphtheria, and pneumonia, and looked at the subjects' immune response to these vaccinations. The researchers also used a skin test that evaluates the overall strength of the immune response.

The results were impressive. Vitamin E at all dosages significantly increased the strength of the immune response. However, a daily dosage of 200 IU produced the most marked benefits.

Although the authors state that their experiment was not really designed to look at whether the number of upper respiratory infections was reduced with use of vitamins, participants were asked to report their own illnesses during the study. A comparison of the participant groups revealed that 74% of the people taking the placebo got some sort of infection, while only 53% of those on vitamin E did. This translates to a significant reduction in infection! However, a study designed specifically to measure this would be necessary to confirm the results. A number of animal studies have already found that vitamin E may offer increased resistance to infection, so this area certainly seems worth investigating.

Dosage

The most common level of vitamin E supplementation is from 200 to 800 IU per day. In the study above, which tested dosages of 60 IU, 200 IU, and 800 IU per day, researchers noted that the best effect was observed at 200 IU daily, and that 800 IU per day did not produce significantly better results. Based on this, we would recommend taking 200 IU of vitamin E daily.

Safety Issues

Vitamin E is believed to be very safe.[6] However, at the high doses used therapeutically, it slightly "thins" the blood. For this reason, high-dose vitamin E should not be combined with drugs such as Coumadin (warfarin) and heparin except on a physician's advice. There might also be risks with weaker blood-thinning substances such as aspirin, ginkgo, and garlic.

Zinc: May Be Beneficial

Another candidate for possible prevention of colds and flus is zinc. See chapter 4 for an explanation about using high-dose zinc lozenges to kill viruses directly in the throat. The basis for using zinc to prevent colds is that zinc is required by the immune system, especially in white blood cells. Zinc deficiency

Zinc and the Ties That Bind

In certain Middle Eastern countries in the early 1960s, an unusually high number of problems were seen among young people involving their growth and sexual development.[10] The cause turned out to be that many people were not getting enough zinc in their diet—not because they weren't eating a lot of foods with zinc in them, but because the zinc was getting "tied up" to other molecules in the grains. Diets in these countries were typically low in meat proteins, and grains were often consumed in the form of unleavened bread. Getting your zinc from shellfish or meats or eating breads prepared with yeast avoids this problem. Yeast, it seems, produces some enzymes that keep more of the zinc free for your body to use.

Although the amount of zinc we need in our daily diet is tiny, it's very important that we get it, as you can see. The evidence, however, suggests that many of us do not get enough. Mild zinc deficiency seems to be fairly common, even in modern, developed countries.

decreases the functioning of t-cells and macrophages.[7,8] Therefore, it seems logical that more zinc might improve their functioning. This may indeed be the case.

Zinc As a Nutritional Supplement

One focus on zinc is its use as a therapeutic agent when taken in very high doses (see chapter 4). Now let's look at it from the perspective of basic nutrition. Zinc is found in every cell we have, and is needed for the enzymes in our bodies to do their life-sustaining work. In short, though we don't need very much zinc, we just can't live without it.

Zinc deficiency can cause a number of physical problems (see the sidebar above); one potential problem is impairment of our immune systems. Surprising as it may seem in this nutrition-conscious society, mild zinc deficiency is fairly common. Children, adolescents, pregnant women, and the elderly are particularly at risk for zinc deficiency; the risk is also greater for those with alcoholism, sickle-cell anemia, and kidney disease. The drug AZT, used for the treatment of AIDS, may impair zinc absorption.[9] The same is true for soy, so if you eat a lot of tofu or drink soy milk, zinc supplements might be a good idea for you.

Oysters are by far the best food source of zinc.

Oysters are by far the best food source of zinc—a single serving will give you 10 times the recommended daily intake! Seeds and nuts, peas, whole wheat, rye, and oats are not nearly as high in zinc, but you can get about 3 mg per serving of these foods.

If you think you might not be getting an adequate amount through your daily food consumption, a supplement might be a good "insurance policy." Zinc citrate, zinc acetate, or zinc picolinate may be the best absorbed, although zinc sulfate is less expensive. See the dosage and safety sections on page 98 for information on safe supplementation with zinc.

Improving Immunity with Zinc

Making sure that you get enough zinc may help reduce the frequency of your colds. In a 2-year study of nursing home residents, participants given 20 mg zinc and 100 mcg of selenium daily developed illnesses much less frequently than those given a placebo.[11]

Of course, it isn't clear from this study which was more helpful, the zinc or the selenium; but because we do know that chronic zinc deficiency weakens the immune system, it seems likely that the increase in zinc would strengthen the immune system.[12]

Furthermore, a 6-month double-blind placebo-controlled study of 609 preschool children in India found that zinc reduced the rate of respiratory infections by 45%.[13]

How Much Zinc Is Enough?

The U.S. Recommended Dietary Allowance for zinc is as follows:

Infants under 1 year	5 mg
Children 1 to 10 years	10 mg
Males 11 years and older	15 mg
Females 11 years and older	12 mg
Pregnant women	15 mg
Nursing women	16 to 19 mg

However, the average diet in the developed world commonly provides less than two-thirds the recommended amount of zinc.[18,19] For this reason, it may be a wise idea to increase your intake of zinc on general principle.

Does zinc help prevent colds only among individuals who are deficient in it? This is not yet clear. However, since zinc deficiency is fairly common, taking it on a "just in case" basis might make sense.

Dosage

To keep your body supplied with enough zinc to stay healthy, simply take the recommended daily requirements listed in the sidebar on page 90. Keep in mind that more isn't better; taking too much zinc can be toxic. (See chapter 4 for safety information, as well as a discussion of high-dose zinc therapy to kill viruses in the throat.)

For best absorption, zinc supplements should not be taken at the same time as high-fiber foods.[14,15] Another factor to keep in mind is that taking vitamins and minerals is sort of a balancing act. (Nutritionists refer to a "balanced" diet with good reason!) When taking zinc long term, you would be well advised to take 1 to 3 mg of copper daily as well, because zinc supplements can cause copper deficiency.[16,17]

Safety Issues

Zinc at the usual recommended dose of 12 to 15 mg is generally considered safe for the long term, provided you follow the advice mentioned above regarding balancing your other minerals, such as copper, iron, and magnesium. For information on safety issues with higher doses of zinc, please see "Safety Issues," page 48.

Vitamin C: May Be Able to Prevent Colds

Research has shown, contrary to popular belief, that taking vitamin C does not prevent colds—*in general.* However, there are a few situations in which it might be helpful.

Some evidence suggests that nutritional doses of vitamin C can decrease the incidence of colds in people who don't get enough vitamin C from their diet.[20] However, if you usually eat your fruits and vegetables, taking C may not help.

A very specific situation in which vitamin C might be useful regards the colds that athletes frequently develop after running a marathon.[21–23]

If you are a marathon runner, you are probably familiar with the "post-race cold," a fairly common phenomenon for those who train for athletic competitions. You train hard for a few weeks before the race to get yourself into shape for peak performance; then you go all out, using up your energy reserves to reach the finish line. Next thing you know, you're lying in bed with the tissues beside you and the vaporizer going full blast, making excuses to your boss on the phone.

Vitamin C might help. According to a double-blind placebo-controlled study involving 92 runners, taking 600 mg of vitamin C for 21 days prior to a race made a significant difference in the incidence of sickness afterwards. While 68% of the runners taking a placebo developed cold symptoms within 2 weeks after the race, only 33% of those taking the vitamin supplement were ill in this time period.

However, as a part of the same study, nonrunners of similar age and gender to those running were also given vitamin C or a placebo. For this group, the vitamin C had no apparent effect on the incidence of upper respiratory infections.

Two other studies involving groups of people involved in heavy exercise also found that vitamin C could reduce the number of colds experienced. Both of these studies used groups of people doing rigorous exercise in extremely cold environments. One study involved 139 children attending a skiing camp in the Swiss Alps, while the other enrolled 56 military men engaged in a training exercise in Northern Canada during the winter months. In both cases, the participants took either 1 g of vitamin C or a placebo daily at the time the training program began. Cold symptoms were monitored for 1 to 2 weeks following training, and significant differences in favor of vitamin C were found.

Vitamin C may protect the immune system from damage caused by free radicals, helping it to fight colds.

However, a third study involving 674 Marine recruits in basic training found no difference in the number of colds between the treatment and placebo groups. Instead of starting the vitamins right at the beginning of training, however, the Marines did not start taking the vitamin C until 3 weeks after they had begun training. The study also lasted a bit longer than the positive studies mentioned above, continuing for 2 months. Otherwise, the study was very similar to the others—leaving vitamin C's effectiveness as a cold preventor somewhat in doubt.

Why Does Vitamin C Seem to Work Only Under Some Conditions?

Several theories make some sense of vitamin C's successes with prevention in conjunction with exercise.[24] Heavy exercise may slow the rate at which certain immune cells are made in our bodies. Perhaps not coincidentally, laboratory studies have found vitamin C to increase the rate at which these same cells are made. Another hand-in-hand observation is that while certain hormones produced during physical stress may depress the immune system, vitamin C may be able to protect immune cells from damage done by these hormones. Heavy exercise is also known to generate damaging types of cells known as free radicals (these were mentioned in chapter 3 as well) that vitamin C, an antioxidant, can neutralize. So taking vitamin C may protect the immune system from damage caused by free radicals, enabling it to better fight off colds. In summary, vitamin C may combat some of the negative effects that exercise can have on our immune system, and thereby prevent infection.

Dosage

The doses used in the studies mentioned above ranged from 600 to 2,000 mg vitamin C daily. We don't know for certain that such large doses are necessary to obtain a protective effect. For more complete information on recommended intake of vitamin C, please see the Dosage section in chapter 3.

Safety Issues

Vitamin C is a very safe supplement. Possible side effects from taking very high doses may include diarrhea, copper deficiency, and excessive iron absorption.

People with a history of kidney stones are advised against taking more than 100 mg of vitamin C daily,[25] and those with glucose-6-phosphate dehydrogenase deficiency (a genetic defect resulting in anemia), iron overload, kidney failure, or a history of intestinal surgery should use vitamin C only under medical supervision.

The maximum safe dosages of vitamin C for young children, pregnant or nursing women, or those with severe liver or kidney disease have not been determined.

For more complete information on the safety of Vitamin C, please see chapter 3.

Lifestyle Changes
for Prevention

H ave you ever dreaded calling in sick . . . *again* . . . knowing that the folks you work for are getting pretty darned tired of your chronic absences? The stress from worrying about how your sick leave is going to affect your job is almost as sickening as your illness! If you get more than your share of colds, flus, and everything else coming down the pike, maybe it's time to consider some lifestyle changes.

If your immune system is functioning normally, you shouldn't get sick every time you come into contact with a communicable disease. You get colds and flus from a combination of your *susceptibility* and *exposure* to illnesses. True, some illnesses are strong enough to make you ill almost every time you come into contact with them. But sometimes a weaker disease gets through and makes you sick because you are just more susceptible at the time.

Many factors contribute to your level of susceptibility. What you eat and drink, where you live and work, your family history, existing medical conditions, travel experiences, and everything else that makes up your daily life have an impact on your immune system. And—hooray!—some of these factors are under your control.

Conditions you can control are your diet, stress level, sleep, exercise, and hygiene. Changes in these areas can and do affect your daily susceptibility to colds and flus, as well as other diseases. Stress is among the most significant of the factors affecting your susceptibility.

Stress

When you think of the word *stress,* perhaps you picture yourself having a really bad day and experiencing negative emotions. Actually, a stressful event can be either negative or positive, psychological or physical.

Traumatic events, such as having a sick relative, a death in the family, or financial troubles, are certainly stressful. Yet so are happy events such as getting married, buying a new home, retiring, or getting a promotion. Less significant occurrences can be stressful, too—for example, not getting enough sleep on a regular basis, taking an exam, getting an annual physical, or driving in heavy traffic. If you simply *perceive* an event as stressful, you'll experience physical and emotional effects of stress in your body.

Reduce the stress you can control, so you can better cope with the stress you can't eliminate.

Stress can be self-propagating—that is, if you're getting sick because your immune system is weakened due to stress, worrying about being sick may create more stress. If you can't sleep because you're "stressed out," the lack of sleep may also contribute to the amount of stress you feel. The good news is that this phenomenon works both ways. Once you break the stress cycle, you can turn a downward spiral into an upward one. Less stress begets less stress.

Stress is not only psychological, but physical. As covered under our discussion of vitamin C in the previous chapter, extremely intense exercise, such as training for and running in a marathon, is known to lower immunity. Endurance athletes frequently get sick after maximal exertion. When we exercise at a highly competitive level, or train intensely for a competitive athletic event, we stress our bodies as we push them to perform.

Stress has many effects on the immune system. For instance, people under stress (including those undergoing medical procedures such as surgery, as one study shows) are more susceptible to infections than other people are.[1] Another study showed that reducing stress improves immunity in people fighting viral infections and even in people with cancer.[2]

While these studies don't signify that stress reduction alone will cure you of disease, they suggest that stress may limit your ability to fight off disease. Stress reduction may therefore be a component of getting better. Long-term or chronic stress is *not* harmless. Reduce the stress you can control, so you can better cope with the stress you can't eliminate.

If you have good coping mechanisms and ways to decrease your stress level, stress won't have as much of an effect on your immune system or the rest of your body. A reasonable amount of regular exercise (for example, half an hour 3 or 4 times per week) helps decrease most people's perception of stress in their lives. Meditation is another popular stress-management tool. Others find that talking with someone about the stressful events in their lives is helpful.

What matters most is how you perceive and handle stress. By taking steps to reduce and manage the stress in your life, you can remove one stumbling block from your immune system's path. Maybe you'll catch one less cold, which in turn means not adding further stress by having to call in sick, which in turn will let your immune system function that much better.

Exercise and Sleep

Exercise and sleep help you live well. At least in part, they may belong in the "Stress" section in terms of how they affect your immune system.

Regular, moderate exercise is like a reset button, clearing away the effects of stress and allowing your body to find its equilibrium. But getting rid of stress is not the only benefit exercise has to offer. When you exercise regularly, you have better circulation of blood, better general health, more energy, and more restful sleep. In addition, as you become more fit, you'll find that you manage some tasks more easily.

Exercise can clear away the effects of stress and allow your body to find its equilibrium.

Lack of sleep is definitely stressful, and most people (rightly) feel that they don't get enough. Sleep experts suggest most people function best on about 8 hours of sleep per night. A 20- to 30-minute nap, in addition to a good night's sleep, can do much toward keeping you healthy and feeling at your best. While you can do your job and live your life on too little sleep, you end up paying the price; fatigue, reduced alertness, and mood swings are classic signs of chronic sleep deprivation. More frequent illness may also follow. So if you're having trouble sleeping, address the problem. Put yourself on a regular sleep schedule, resist picking up that murder mystery right at bedtime, or switch to decaf in the afternoon. Try some of the methods covered above for reducing stress—exercise, meditation, talking about your worries—so that you can get some sleep. Your body will thank you.

Nutrition

Your diet definitely affects your immune system, as well as the rest of your body. What you do (and do not) eat can make you more or less susceptible to illness. People suffering from vitamin and mineral malnutrition often have more than their share of infections.

Eating well can help your immune system function optimally. Make sure you're eating a balanced diet and getting

Table 1. Vitamins and Minerals Needed
for a Healthy Immune System

Vitamin or Mineral	RDA for Adults	Immune System Effects
Zinc[3]	12 to 15 mg	Proper function of white blood cells, especially T-lymphocytes and macrophages
Vitamin A	4,000 to 5,000 IU	T- and B-lymphocyte responses to antigens; may help phagocytosis
B complex[4–7]		
B1 (thiamin)	1 to 1.5 mg	Proper antibody response to antigens
B2 (riboflavin)	1.2 to 1.8 mg	
B5 (pantothenic acid)	4 to 7 mg	
B6	1.5 to 2 mg	
B12	2 mcg	
Vitamin E[8–10]	12 to 15 IU	Lymphocyte production and function
Copper[11,12]	No RDA (safe and adequate range is 1.5 to 3 mg)	Normal function of lymphocytes and the bacteria-killing abilities of granulocytes

enough vitamins and minerals, as well as adequate protein. The vitamins and minerals that are important to proper functioning and maintenance of the immune system are listed in table 1.

Protein deficiency, like vitamin and mineral deficiencies, can suppress your immune system, and studies also show that deficiencies in other nutrients such as essential fatty acids can decrease your body's ability to react to antigens. People with anorexia or bulimia often suffer from malnutrition and may experience immune deficiency as a result, especially because of deficiencies of protein, vitamins, and minerals. Protein deficiency

Was Grandma Right about That Sweater?

According to folk tradition, getting chilled causes colds. Certainly people seem to catch more colds and flus when the weather turns wintry, but we don't know why. One theory holds that cold weather stimulates the flow of mucus, which may provide a good place for viruses to grow; but whether this situation actually contributes to the frequency of viral infections in humans is unknown. Another frequently stated explanation clearly has some truth to it: People tend to congregate more closely in the winter months, giving viruses a better opportunity to spread. You tend to be closer to other people all day long (who wants to eat lunch outside in the winter?) in a closed environment where others are sneezing and coughing. This situation helps transmit the viruses that remain floating in the air you breathe. As well, you will spend more time breathing *that* air instead of outdoor air, in which viruses tend to disperse.

Furthermore, you are likely to experience more physical shock from major temperature changes as you move between the cold outdoors and heated buildings. (This shock happens in the summer, too, as you go from the outside heat into air-conditioned cars and buildings.) Exposure to sudden temperature changes may in some way weaken your immunity. Top it off with the stress of the holidays and the fact that you may be unable to get outside to practice your favorite form of exercise, and you may well get sick.

can also occur in people who are dieting or who restrict what they eat for other reasons. People who consume adequate calories may still fail to get enough protein. For example, vegetarians who fail to educate themselves on how to eat a healthful, balanced vegetarian diet may suffer from protein deficiency.

It does take a little extra time to pay attention to what you're putting in your body. However, if you spend more time making salads, you're likely to spend less time blowing your

---

And You Thought You Knew
How to Wash Your Hands . . .

If your mom admonished you to wash both the front and back of your hands when you were a kid, she was right—but that is not enough. Many people wash their hands in less than 10 seconds, and some never bother to use soap. A good hand washing takes 30 seconds and involves soap on all surfaces of the hands. You should lather thoroughly and rinse with your fingers down, so the water flows from your wrists to fingers. Finally, don't turn off the water (which you turned on with your dirty hands) with your newly clean hands. Get a paper towel from the dispenser, or get a tissue at home, and use that to touch the handle and turn off the water.

---

nose. Isn't that time well spent? After all, nothing is more important than taking good care of yourself.

Other Factors You Can Control

If the recommendations in the previous sections sound like your mother talking ("Get a good night's sleep, and remember to eat your vegetables!"), brace yourself. Mom had even more good advice.

Hand Washing

It seems so basic, but proper hand washing is an important step in preventing colds and flus. We all know about washing our hands after we go to the bathroom or before and after handling food, but few of us think much about hand washing at other times.

Colds and flus are spread through secretions from the mouth, throat, and nasal passages. These secretions can easily be passed from person to person, especially between those in close contact. A sneeze or cough will spread the virus into the air or onto the hand or handkerchief of the person who sneezed or coughed. You might inhale the virus from the air, but you might also pick it up on your hands from a surface such as a telephone recently touched by someone with the virus on their hands. If you take care of someone who has a cold or flu, you constantly touch surfaces on which the virus has settled. Although these viruses don't live long outside the human body, they can survive long enough for you to pick them up and transfer them to your own eyes, mouth, or nose. Frequently washing your hands helps prevent the viruses from taking advantage of the opportunity to invade your body.

If the bad news is that these viruses continually get onto your hands during cold and flu season, the good news is that your skin is a pretty good barrier. You don't get sick simply by touching someone who has a cold or flu or by touching something they have touched. You get sick when the virus actually makes contact with the mucous membranes that line your mouth and nose (your susceptibility is a factor as well). However, unconsciously wiping your nose or mouth can take the viruses right to their favorite point of entry.

The bottom line is that you need to wash your hands frequently, probably more than you normally do. You don't need to rush to the bathroom or to expensive "water-free" hand cleaners every time you touch something that someone else touched first. You do need to wash your hands before eating; before touching your mouth, eyes, or nose; and after being in close contact with someone who has a cold or flu. If you're taking care of someone who is infected, make sure she covers her mouth and nose when she sneezes or coughs—health-care professionals recommend teaching children to use the crook of an elbow instead of their hands, to avoid smearing the germs all over whatever they touch next.

Even so, wash your hands after you touch surfaces or objects a cold sufferer has handled—especially those used tissues—and every time you leave the sickroom!

Drinking

Mom might have wanted you to stay out of the bars for other reasons, but avoiding excessive intake of alcohol and smoke (your own or someone else's) will probably help you avoid down-time with flus and colds as well. If you didn't believe your mother, listen to your doctor, who will probably tell you the same thing. Smoking, especially, is associated with greater susceptibility to colds.[13]

Food Sensitivities

Many alternative practitioners feel that food sensitivities play a part in our daily susceptibility to illness, as well as to other conditions. The theory is that you may have a low-level sensitivity to certain foods, a condition similar but not necessarily identical to an allergy. This sensitivity may cause enough disturbance to the body to increase susceptibility to infection.

Some individuals do appear to benefit from eliminating certain foods from their diets. Unfortunately, performing double-blind studies on diet is next to impossible (since it's obvious whether or not you're eating cheese, for example). For this reason, discovering just what role, if any, food sensitivities play in health and illness is difficult.

What you do (and do not) eat can make you more or less susceptible to illness.

If you are aware that certain foods don't agree with you, try avoiding them when you get your next cold to see whether you feel better. Some of the most common foods mentioned as problematic besides milk are wheat, sugar, and caffeine-containing foods.[14–18] Avoiding these foods for a week or two to see whether they affect your body poses little risk. You can also try eliminating these foods for a long period of time and see whether doing so reduces the number of colds you develop. If you restrict your diet for a long time, however, you may suffer from malnutrition. Malnutrition can decrease immunity, and eliminating too many foods can cause malnutrition.

If you are interested in a major diet overhaul, see a physician who can help you make sure you still get enough of all the essential nutrients. This is especially important for children, whose growing bodies require excellent nutrition.

Aging and Immunity

We can't avoid every factor that influences the strength of our immune systems. One unavoidable factor is aging. While aging is not, in and of itself, always a state of decline, some aspects of our health typically do decline as we age. Biological changes inevitably take place as we get older, and many of these start when we are in our 30s. Humans in their 30s are different than they were during their teen years, and they change even more by the time they reach their 50s.

While we don't understand the mechanisms or reasons for most of the changes that occur with age, we are becoming more familiar with the changes themselves. For instance, we know that a decrease in bone marrow occurs. Bone marrow makes all our blood cells, so the older we get, the less we can respond to the need for more white blood cells (or more red cells, for that matter). It doesn't mean we can't make them, just that we have less bone marrow to do the job for us.

This makes it all the more important, as the years go by, to pay closer attention to those things we can control—diet, exercise, stress reduction, and so forth. And if taking vitamins and perhaps an herbal supplement can help us level out the playing field, why not take advantage of that?

CHAPTER

T E N

Medications for Colds and Flus

S ince the 1940s, herbal medicine has been out of favor with conventional medicine in the United States. Perhaps as a result of this, many people think of herbs and vitamins as being less powerful than conventional medicine. This, however, depends on the drug and the herb being compared, and on the particular use. The treatment of colds and flus is a good example of a situation in which natural treatments may in some cases prove more effective than standard medications. While echinacea, zinc, andrographis, and other herbs and supplements appear to shorten the duration of colds, standard "cold care" medications only relieve symptoms, if they even do that. Medications that lessen the symptoms of flus don't seem much different in effectiveness from echinacea, elderberry, or andrographis.

In this chapter, we'll cover therapies offered by pharmaceutical companies for colds and flus, available either on the aisles of your local drugstore or in the pharmacy by prescription from your doctor.

If you're like most people, you've probably spent your share of time in the cold and flu aisle of the pharmacy. There are a *lot* of products from which to choose—for your sore throat, your stuffy head, your aches and fever, and for combinations of these

Visit Us at TNP.com

and other symptoms. But as we mentioned back in chapter 1, these over-the-counter medications are only good for symptom management; they won't rid your body of the virus that's making you sick, and they can't help your immune system fight off the virus.

Some prescription medications can help prevent or shorten the duration of the flu if you take them early enough, but no medication as yet can help you avoid the common cold. Similarly, while you can get a shot to ward off some flus, no effective vaccine is available to prevent the common cold. But let's talk a bit about what vaccines *can* (and can't) do.

Using Vaccines to Prevent the Flu

You develop immunity from being exposed to a virus, bacteria, or anything your body sees as a dangerous invader. Medical science refers to invaders that evoke such a response from your body as *antigens*. Your body reacts by making antibodies and white blood cells that recognize and attack the particular "enemy." Some of these cells remain in your body after you get well, and their presence speeds up your immune response the next time you encounter the same antigen. You may not get sick at all on a repeat exposure and are unlikely ever to get as sick as you did the first time you encountered that antigen.

Over-the-counter medications are good only for symptom management.

Immunizations, also known as vaccinations, work on this principle. Here's how vaccinations make you immune to diseases you've never caught: You are exposed (usually via injection) to a very small amount of an antigen, such as a weakened virus. Your body then produces antibodies and white blood cells specific to this antigen. The next time you encounter that antigen, either through another immunization or "in the wild" (meaning from someone who is actually sick with the disease caused by the antigen—measles, for example), your immune system responds more quickly and efficiently, eliminating the antigen before you actually get sick. This happens because the first exposure via vaccination gives your immune system a head start so you can quickly produce lots of antibodies and lymphocytes to work against that antigen.

Unfortunately, in the case of the common cold, no vaccine is available, mostly because so many different viruses can cause a cold. Vaccinating against every virus that causes colds has proven impossible thus far.

For the flu, however, you can protect yourself with a relatively effective vaccine. Each year, the flu vaccine is made from the strain of flu that circulated the year before. How well the

Vaccinating against colds has proven impossible, but you can protect yourself from flus with a relatively effective vaccine.

shot will protect you varies, depending on how similar the vaccine is to the virus circulating and how well your body normally fights off diseases. If the virus that was "grown" in the laboratory to make the vaccine is a whole lot like the one infecting people out on the streets, up to 80% of the people who got a flu shot will manage to avoid the flu entirely.[1] Those who don't escape it entirely will typically have many fewer complications and less severe cases of the flu than unvaccinated people. Keep in mind that the herb ginseng may augment the benefits of the flu vaccine (see chapter 7).

The vaccine is a good preventive measure for those in groups at high risk for exposure and for exposing others— health-care workers and school teachers, for example. Vaccination is also recommended for those at greater risk for serious complications, such as elderly people or those with lowered immune responses.

However, if you already have the flu, the vaccine won't do you a bit of good. So what does conventional medicine have to offer if you already feel symptoms coming on?

Antiviral Drugs for the Flu

Two drugs, amantadine and rimantadine, are commonly used to lessen the ugliness of your flu (technically, influenza A) once you're already sick. These medications can decrease the duration and severity of your illness—but only if you take them within the first 48 hours after you develop symptoms. These drugs can also be used for prevention, so if someone in your house or at work has the flu, you could benefit by visiting your doctor early and asking about these medications. Your physician might be willing to provide a prescription for either amantadine or rimantadine for you to have on hand at the beginning of flu season, since both are relatively safe.

Rimantadine and amantadine appear to make it harder for a virus to multiply by interfering with a process called "uncoating," one of the first steps the virus has to go through to make copies of itself. This gives your immune system a chance to gear up before it must fight against untold trillions of the virus. These medications are usually taken for a course of 10 days if you have the flu yourself. During that time, you should rest and avoid exposing other people to your flu. You may not feel truly awful, but you still have the flu. If you use one of these drugs for prevention, you'll want to keep taking it as long as your coworker, children, or whoever has the flu remains ill and in contact with you.

A new drug has just been approved by the FDA for treatment of both influenza A and B.

Rimantadine is more commonly used than amantadine because it is equally effective but has fewer side effects. Amantadine works, but some people who take it (5% to 10%) have side effects such as anxiety, jitteriness, insomnia, and difficulty concentrating. These drugs are safe for most people, and are generally effective in managing uncomplicated cases of the flu.

In addition, a new drug called zanamivir (sold as Relenza) was recently approved by the FDA for treatment of both influenza A and B. Evidence suggests it can shorten your 7-day flu by about 1 to 2 days.[2] Furthermore, the drug seems to be about 80% effective at preventing flus among other family members when one member has come down with it.

Like rimantadine and amantadine, zanamivir has to be used when the flu is in its early stages. Unlike rimantadine and amantadine, the new drug comes in the form of a nasal spray or inhaler, not in pill form. It works by inhibiting enzymes needed by the influenza viruses.

The Pharmacy Shelf

Besides the treatments your doctor can prescribe for flu prevention and control, many over-the-counter medications are available for treating the symptoms of colds and flus. Most likely you've sampled them at some point, and perhaps you already know they help with your symptoms to some extent, but don't help you get well any quicker. The virus is still replicating in your cells, and you'll just have to wait until your immune system has the situation under control before you really feel like yourself again. Probably the most effective over-the-counter cold and flu treatments are pain relievers and fever reducers, such as acetaminophen, aspirin, ibuprofen, and naproxen. They can significantly reduce the muscle aches and headache pain of the flu and may somewhat relieve the discomfort of a head cold.

The decongestants pseudoephedrine and phenylpropanolamine may help relieve sinus discomfort, but they can also cause restlessness and insomnia, and might increase blood pressure.

The expectorant guaifenesin, included in many cough syrups and a few pills, can help break up thick mucus. Dextromethorphan

Superbugs and Chicken Feed

Many people—including some doctors—appear to regard the warnings about overuse of antibiotics as hearsay. Regrettably, these warnings are based upon a growing body of evidence. The number of antibiotic-resistant bacteria, or "superbugs," has increased dramatically over the last two decades, and the reason is thought to be the casual use of antibiotics.

In May of 1999, the Centers for Disease Control reported an alarming increase in the numbers of antibiotic-resistant types of salmonella, a bacterium that causes severe food poisoning, and sometimes death. Of all the samples tested in the United States for resistance in 1980, 0.6% could not be killed by any of five different antibiotics. In 1996, 34% were resistant to the same group of antibiotics.[3]

How did this happen? One of the culprits is the practice of feeding antibiotics to animals raised for human consumption along with their feed on a daily basis. When bacteria multiply, a small number may develop resistance to an antibiotic. When the antibiotic is present, those that have no resistance are killed, leaving much more space for the resistant bacteria to grow and thrive. Feeding the same antibiotics used for treating human disease to barnyard animals is much like setting up a factory to create infections we can't control.

is also a common ingredient in cough syrups. It suppresses a cough and is best used at night to help you sleep.

Antihistamines such as chlorpheniramine and tripolidine are often found in cold remedies, but neither is of much use in colds, except to help you fall asleep. Combination cold remedies contain many of these ingredients mixed together, frequently along with alcohol, but you will often do better by taking just the ingredients you need.

Better still, you might want to try some of the supplements that not only reduce the severity of your symptoms, but might

The newest antibiotic drug, Zyvox, has not yet been approved for use by the FDA.[4] If it is sanctioned for human use, it should provide doctors with a new weapon to combat resistant organisms—for a while. However, laboratory testing has already revealed three cases of resistance to Zyvox before it hits the market.

Synercid, an antibiotic that has already run the FDA's gauntlet and won approval, is one of a class of drugs that has already been used for years in animal feeds in Europe—meaning it's a very good bet that Synercid-resistant bacteria either already exist or lurk right around the corner.

Overuse of antibiotics to treat human patients allows resistant organisms to develop in people in exactly the same way. Taking such drugs when you have a viral infection does nothing to treat your illness, and allows drug-resistant organisms to begin colonizing you, personally.

To avoid becoming a walking "superbug" factory, let your doctor know that you only want antibiotics if there is good reason to believe that you are suffering from a bacterial infection. To get relief from the average flu or cold, you may want to try one of the herbs or supplements that has been found to really help with viral illness, such as zinc or andrographis.

also help you get over the cold sooner, such as zinc, vitamin C, echinacea, and others.

Antibiotics

Contrary to popular belief, antibiotics are not useful for colds and flus. Antibiotics kill bacteria, not viruses. In the past, people often died of bacterial infections such as bacterial pneumonia and plague, which we now easily treat with antibiotics. However, antibiotics are completely ineffective against colds and flus, which are caused by viruses. You'd be more likely to get results using zinc lozenges, which may be able to kill or at least inhibit cold viruses in the throat (see chapter 4 for more details).

Despite the fact that antibiotics don't kill viruses, people often go to the doctor and insist that they need antibiotics—and sometimes get them—for the treatment of common viral infections. These patients may even claim that the antibiotics help (although what they are experiencing is probably the placebo effect). This misuse of antibiotics has contributed to the development of "superbugs," bacteria that are resistant to many or even all antibiotics.

The only cases in which antibiotics are appropriate for colds are those in which a person initially infected with a viral infection *also* develops a bacterial infection. Medical authorities strongly recommend (and even beg!) doctors and patients to limit antibiotic use to situations in which antibiotics are truly necessary, but getting people to cooperate is difficult.

Sometimes doctors assume that patients will insist on antibiotics, so prescribe them as a matter of course. By telling your doctor that you want antibiotics only when absolutely necessary, you'll be doing your part to keep these vital drugs effective when they are truly needed.

CHAPTER
ELEVEN

Putting It All Together

H ere we'll briefly summarize the natural treatments described throughout this book. Please refer to the respective chapters for a more detailed discussion of each treatment, including information on dosage and safety issues.

There are two ways to use natural treatments for colds and flus. Some treatments can be taken at the onset of symptoms to help you get over the infection more rapidly and feel less sick during the process; others can be taken regularly to reduce the chance of getting sick in the first place.

Note: If your physician has recommended that you get a flu shot, do not try to use natural treatments as a substitute.

Natural Treatments for Your Colds and Flus

There is evidence that certain herbs and supplements—such as echinacea, andrographis, zinc, and vitamin C—may reduce the length of time you are sick, as well as the severity of your symptoms.

Good evidence tells us that **echinacea** can reduce the severity and duration of colds and flus. Take it at the first sign of illness, and continue for 7 to 14 days. The typical dosage of echinacea powdered extract is 300 mg 3 times a day. Alcohol tincture (1:5) is usually taken at a dosage of 3 to 4 ml 3 times daily, echinacea juice at a dosage of 2 to 3 ml 3 times daily, and whole dried root at 1 to 2 g 3 times daily. Some formulas may require different dosing, so read the label carefully. Echinacea is generally quite safe, although certain considerations apply in special situations.

Vitamin C, according to clinical studies, can reduce cold symptoms and slightly improve recovery time. A typical recommended dose for use at the onset of colds is 500 mg 3 times a day. For more information on dosage and safety, see chapter 3.

Research findings indicated that **zinc lozenges** can help you get over a cold significantly more quickly. At the first sign of infection, begin sucking lozenges containing 13.3 to 23 mg of zinc as zinc gluconate or zinc acetate, 1 every 2 hours while awake. Flavorings may affect lozenge effectiveness, as described in chapter 4. Zinc should not be used for more than 2 weeks at these therapeutic doses (see the Dosage and Safety sections in chapter 4).

A few studies suggest that the herb **andrographis** can be helpful for colds. A typical dose of andrographis is 400 mg 3 times a day, standardized to 4 to 6% andrographolide. See chapter 5 for information on safety.

Among the less-researched substances, **elderberry** extract was found in one small clinical trial to shorten the duration of flus. Standardized extract should be taken according to the manufacturer's recommendations.

Other less-researched alternatives, including osha, mullein, peppermint, yerba santa, marshmallow, kudzu, ginger, yarrow, and garlic, have been suggested by some for treating colds and flus, but no clinical studies support this. Goldenseal has neither historic tradition nor scientific evidence to support its use for this purpose.

Preventing Colds and Flus

A number of herbs and supplements are said to be able to ward off colds and flus.

A class of herbs called *adaptogens* is widely believed to strengthen immunity. Several medicinal plants are thought to have these qualities, including ginseng, *Eleutherococcus* ("Siberian ginseng"), astragalus, ashwagandha, maitake, reishi, and suma, but *Panax ginseng* (Asian ginseng) is the best researched.

In one study, **ginseng** was found to enhance the effects of a flu vaccine and significantly reduce infections. The typical dose is 100 to 200 mg of standardized ginseng extract (standardized to 4 to 7% ginsenosides) daily.

Other herbs and supplements may also aid in prevention. Andrographis, vitamin E, zinc, and vitamin C may help keep colds and flus away, although vitamin C's benefits are only seen under certain conditions.

Andrographis at 200 mg daily, standardized to 5.6% andrographolide, may increase resistance to colds. See chapter 8 for more information on dosage and safety.

Vitamin E significantly increased the strength of the immune response in one study and also appeared to reduce the number of flu infections the participants experienced. A daily dosage of 200 IU produced the most marked benefits.

Taking zinc supplements long term at a daily dose of 12 to 15 mg may help reduce the frequency of your colds if you are deficient in this mineral. Higher doses of zinc can cause toxicity over time. For information on safety issues, see the Safety sections for zinc in chapters 4 and 8.

Nutritional doses of vitamin C may decrease the incidence of colds in people who habitually run short on this vitamin. It has also been found to be helpful for preventing colds that develop following periods of physical stress, such as training for athletic events. Possible side effects with very high doses may include diarrhea, copper deficiency, and excessive iron absorption. For complete information, see the Dosage and Safety sections for vitamin C in chapter 8.

Notes

About Colds and Flus

1. Schulz V, et al. *Rational phytotherapy*. 3rd ed. New York: Springer-Verlag; 1998:246.

Echinacea: The Most Famous Herb for Colds

1. Bone K. Echinacea: What makes it work? *Altern Med Rev.* 1997;2(2):87–93.

2. Schulz V, et al. *Rational phytotherapy*. 3rd ed. New York: Springer-Verlag; 1998:278.

3. Melchart D, et al. Immunomodulation with echinacea: a systematic review of controlled clinical trials. *Phytomedicine.* 1994;1:245–254.

4. Brinkeborn RM, et al. Echinaforce and other echinacea fresh plant preparations in the treatment of the common cold. A randomized, placebo controlled, double-blind clinical trial. *Phytomedicine.* 1999;6(1):1–5.

5. Braunig B, et al. *Echinacea purpurea* radix for strengthening the immune response in flu-like infections. *Z Phytother.* 1992;13:7–13.

6. Dorn M, et al. Placebo-controlled, double-blind study of *Echinaceae pallidae* radix in upper respiratory tract infections. *Complement Ther Med.* 1997;3:40–42.

7. Dorn M. Milderung grippaler Effekte durch ein pflanzliches Immunstimulans. *Natur und Ganzheitsmedizin.* 1989;2:314–319.

8. Hoheisel O, et al. Echinagard treatment shortens the course of the common cold: a double-blind placebo-controlled clinical trial. *Eur J Clin Res.* 1997;9:261–268.

9. Coeugniet E, Kuhnhast R. Recurrent candidiasis: adjuvant immunotherapy with different formulations of Echinacin Æ. *Therapiewoche.* 1986;36:3352–3358.

10. Tubaro A, et al. Anti-inflammatory activity of a polysaccharidic fraction of *Echinacea angustifolia. J Pharm Pharmacol.* 1987;39(7):567.

11. Muller-Jakic B, et al. In vitro inhibition of cyclooxygenase and 5-lipoxygenase by alkamides from *Echinacea* and *Achillea* species. *Planta Med.* 1994;60(1):37.

12. Tragni E, et al. Antiinflammatory activity *of Echinacea angustifolia* fractions separated on the basis of molecular weight. *Pharmacol Res Commun.* 1988;20(suppl 5):87.

13. Busing KH. Inhibition of hyaluronidase by echinacin. *Arzneimittelforschung.* 1952;2:467–469.

14. Busing KH. Hyaluronidase inhibition of some naturally occurring substances used in therapy. *Arzneimittelforschung.* 1955; 5:320–322.

15. Coeugniet E, Kuhnhast R. Recurrent candidiasis: adjuvant immunotherapy with different formulations of Echinacin Æ. *Therapiewoche.* 1986;36:3352–3358.

16. Jurcic K, et al. Zwei Probandenstudien zur Stimulierung durch Echinacea-Extrakt-haltige Praparate. *Z Phytother.* (English abstract only). 1989;10:67–70.

17. Bauer R, et al. *Z Phytother.* 1989;10:43.

18. Vomel T. Einfluss eines unspezifischen immunstimulans auf die phagozytose von erthrozyten und tusche durch das retikulohistiozytare system unterschiedlich alter, isolert perfundierter rattenlebern (English abstract only). *Arzneimittelforschung/Drug Res.* 1984;34:691–695.

19. Bauer VR, et al. Immunologische in vivo und in vitro unterschungen mit echinacea-extrakten (English abstract only). *Arzneimittelforschung/Drug Res.* 1988;38:276–281.

20. Gaisbauer M, et al. Untersuchungen zum einflub von echinacea purpurea moench auf die phagozytose von granulozyten mittels messung der chemilumineszenz (English abstract only). *Arzneimittel-forschung/Drug Res.* 1990;40:594–598.

21. Wagner H, Proksch A. An immunostimulating active principal from *Echinacea purpurea* Moench. *Z Angew Phytother.* 1981;2(5):166–168.

22. Stimpel M, et al. Macrophage activation and induction of macrophage cytotoxicity by purified polysaccharide fraction of the plant *Echinacea purpurea. Infect Immun.* 1984;46(3):845–849.

23. Luettig B, et al. Macrophage activation by the polysaccharide arabinogalactan isolated from plant cell cultures of *Echinacea purpurea. J Nat Cancer Inst.* 1989;81(9):669–675.

24. Snow JM. *Echinacea* (Moench) spp. Asteraceae. *Protocol J Bot Med.* 1997;2(2):18–24.

25. Bauer R, Wagner H. Echinacea species as potential immunostimulatory drugs. *Econ Med Plant Res.* 1991;5:253–321.

26. Bone K. 1997.

27. Heinzer F, et al. Classification of the therapeutically used species of the genus Echinacea. *Pharm Acta Helv.* 1988;63(4–5):132–136.

28. Wagner H, Proksch A. 1981.

29. Stimpel M, et al. Macrophage activation and induction of macrophage cytotoxicity by purified polysaccharide fraction of the plant *Echinacea purpurea. Infect Immun.* 1984;46(3):845–849.

30. Luettig B, et al. Macrophage activation by the polysaccharide arabinogalactan isolated from plant cell cultures of *Echinacea purpurea. J Nat Cancer Inst.* 1989;81(9):669–675.

31. Bone K. 1997.

32. Bauer R, et al. Immunological in vivo and in vitro examinations of echinacea extracts. *Arzneimittelforschung.* 1988;38(2):276–281.

33. Bergner P. Goldenseal and the common cold: The antibiotic myth. *Med Herbalism.* 1997;8(4):1–10.

34. Schulz V, et al. 1998.

35. Mengs U, et al. Toxicity of *Echinacea purpurea* acute, subacute, and genotoxicity studies. *Arzneimittelforschung/Drug Res.* 1991;41(11):1076–1081.

36. Parnham MJ. Benefit-risk assessment of the squeezed sap of the purple coneflower *(Echinacea purpurea)* for long-term oral immunostimulation. *Phytomedicine.* 1996;3(1):99–102.

37. Becker H, Hsieh WC. Cichoric acid and its derivatives from *Echinacea* species. *Z Naturforsch C: Biosci.* 1985;40C(7–8):585–587.

38. Facino R, Meffei M. Direct characterization of caffeoyl esters with antihyaluronidase activity in crude extracts from *Echinacea angustifolia* roots by fast atom bombardment tandem mass spectrometry. *Farmaco.* 1993;48(10):1447–1461.

39. Snow JM. 1997.

40. Bone K. 1997.

Vitamin C: A Cold-and-Flu Treatment Contender

1. Hemilä H. Does vitamin C alleviate symptoms of the common cold? A review of current evidence. *Scand J Infect Dis.* 1994;26:1–6.

2. Hemilä H. Vitamin C and the common cold. *Br J Nutr.* 1992;67:3–16.

3. Chalmers TC. Effects of ascorbic acid on the common cold. An evaluation of the evidence. *Am J Med.* 1975;58:532–536.

4. Hemilä H, et al. Vitamin C and the common cold: a retrospective analysis of Chalmers' review. *J Am Coll Nutr.* 1995;14:116–123.

5. Hemilä H. Vitamin C intake and susceptibility to the common cold. *Br J Nutr.* 1997;77:1–14.

6. Hemilä H. 1992.

7. Hercberg S, et al. Vitamin status of a healthy French population: dietary intakes and biochemical markers. *Int J Vitam Nutr Res.* 1994;64(3):220–232.

8. Lowik MR, et al. Assessment of the adequacy of vitamin C intake in the Netherlands. (abstract). *J Am Coll Nutr.* 1991;10(5):544.

9. U.S. Department of Agriculture. *National Food Consumption Survey.* 1985.

10. Baker B. Vitamin C deficiency common in hospitalized. *Fam Pract News.* March 15, 1995;25.

11. Holt GA. *Food and Drug Interactions.* Chicago: Precept Press; 1998:83.

12. Coffey G, Wilson SWM. Letter: Ascorbic acid deficiency and aspirin-induced haematemesis. *Br Med J.* 1975;1:208.

13. Hodges R. Drug-nutrient interaction. Cited by: Hodges R. *Nutrition in Medical Practice.* Philadelphia: W.B. Saunders; 1980:323–331.

14. Holt GA. 1998.

15. Levine M, et al. Vitamin C pharmacokinetics in health volunteers: evidence for a recommended dietary allowance. *Proc Natl Acad Sci USA.* 1996;93(8)3704–3709.

16. Austin S. Vitamin C and mutagenesis—much ado about nothing? *Q Rev Nat Med.* Portland, OR: HealthNotes, Inc; Fall 1998;227.

17. Auer BL, et al. Relative hyperoxaluria, crystalluria, and hematuria after mega-dose ingestion of vitamin C. *Eur J Clin Invest.* 1998;28:695–700.

18. Levine M, et al. 1996.

19. Curhan GC, et al. A prospective study of the intake of vitamins C and B6 and the risk of kidney stones in men. *J Urol.* 1996;155:1847–51.

20. Gerster H. No contribution of ascorbic acid to renal calcium oxalate stones. *Ann Nutr Metab.* 1997;41:269–282.

21. Auer BL, et al. Relative hyperoxaluria, crystalluria, and hematuria after mega-dose ingestion of vitamin C. *Eur J Clin Invest.* 1998;28:695–700.

22. Owen CA Jr., et al. Heparin-ascorbic acid antagonism. *Mayo Clin Proc.* 1970;45:140.

23. Rosenthal G. Interaction of ascorbic acid and warfarin. *JAMA.* 1971;215:1671.

24. Harris JE. Interaction of dietary factors with oral anticoagulants: Review and applications. *J Am Dietet Assoc.* 1995;95:580–4.

25. Hankinson S, et al. Nutrient intake and cataract extraction in women: a prospective study. *BMJ.* 1992;305:335–339.

26. Jacques PF, et al. Long-term vitamin C supplement use and prevalence of early age-related lens opacities. *Am J Clin Nutr.* 1997;66:911–916.

27. Will JC, et al. Does diabetes mellitus increase the requirement for vitamin C? *Nutr Rev.* 1996;54:193–202.

28. Mares-Perlman J, et al. Relationship between age-related maculopathy and intake of vitamin and mineral supplements (abstract). *Invest Ophthalmol Vis Sci.* 1993;34:1133.

29. Mares-Perlman JA, et al. Association of zinc and antioxidant nutrients with age-related maculopathy. *Arch Ophthalmol.* 1996;114:991–997.

30. Age-Related Macular Degeneration Study Group. Multicenter ophthalmic and nutritional age-related macular degeneration study—Part 2: antioxidant intervention and conclusions. *J Am Optom Assoc.* 1996;67:30–49.

31. Taylor TV, et al. Ascorbic acid supplementation in the treatment of pressure-sores. *Lancet.* 1974;2:544–546.

32. Dawson EB, et al. Effect of ascorbic acid on male fertility. *Ann N Y Acad Sci.* 1987;498:312–323.

33. Bielory L, Gandhi R. Asthma and vitamin C. *Ann Allergy.* 1994;73:89–96.

34. Osilesi O, et al. Blood pressure and plasma lipids during ascorbic acid supplementation in borderline hypertensive and normotensive adults. *Nutr Res.* 1991;11:405–412.

35. Feldman E, et al. Ascorbic acid supplements and blood pressure. *Ann N Y Acad Sci.* 1992;669:342–344.

36. Ghosh S, Ekpo E, Shah I. A double-blind, placebo-controlled parallel trial of vitamin C treatment in elderly patients with hypertension. *Gerontology.* 1994;40:268–272.

37. McAlindon TE, et al. Do antioxidant micronutrients protect against the development and progression of knee OA? *Arthritis Rheum.* 1996;39:648–656.

38. Schwartz ER. The modulation of osteoarthritic development by vitamins C and E. *Int J Vit Nutr Res Suppl.* 1984;26:141–146.

39. Cameron E, Pauling L. Supplemental ascorbate in the supportive treatment of cancer: prolongation of survival times in terminal human cancer. *Proc Natl Acad Sci USA.* 1976;73:3685–3689.

40. Cameron E, Campbell A. Innovation vs. quality control: an "unpublishable" clinical trial of supplemental ascorbate in incurable cancer. *Med Hypotheses.* 1991;36:185–189.

41. Creagan ET, et al. Failure of high-dose vitamin C (ascorbic acid) therapy to benefit patients with advanced cancer. A controlled trial. *N Engl J Med.* 1979;301:687–690.

42. Moertel CG, et al. High-dose vitamin C versus placebo in the treatment of patients with advanced cancer who have had no prior chemotherapy. A randomized double-blind comparison. *N Engl J Med.* 1985;312:137–141.

Zinc for Colds and Flus

1. Marshall S. Zinc gluconate and the common cold. Review of randomized controlled trials. *Can Fam Physician.* 1998;44:1037–1042.

2. Girodon F, et al. Effect of micronutrient supplementation on infection in institutionalized elderly subjects: a controlled trial. *Ann Nutr Metab.* 1997;41(2):98–107.

3. Marshall S. 1998.

4. Eby GA. Linearity in dose-response from zinc lozenges in treatment of common colds. *J Pharmacy Technol.* 1995;11:110–122.

5. Eby GA. Zinc ion availability—the determinant of efficacy in zinc lozenge treatment of common colds. *J Antimicrob Chemother.* 1997;40:483–493.

6. Mossad SB, et al. Zinc gluconate lozenges for treating the common cold: a randomized, double-blind placebo-controlled study. *Ann Intern Med.* 1996;125:142–144.

7. Marshall S. 1998.

8. Eby GA. 1997.

9. Macknin ML, et al. Zinc gluconate lozenges for treating the common cold in children: a randomized controlled trial. *JAMA.* 1998;279:1962–1967.

10. Petrus EJ, Lawson KA, Bucci LR. Randomized, double-masked, placebo-controlled clinical study of the effectiveness of zinc acetate lozenges on common cold symptoms in allergy-tested subjects. *Curr Ther Res.* 1998;59:595–607.

11. Marshall S. 1998.

12. Eby GA. 1997.

13. Petrus EJ, Lawson KA, Bucci LR. 1998.

14. Eby GA. 1997.

15. Eby GA. 1997.

16. Hoffman HN II, et al. Zinc-induced copper deficiency. *Gastro-enterology.* 1988;94:508–512.

17. Sandstead HH. Requirements and toxicity of essential trace elements, illustrated by zinc and copper. *Am J Clin Nutr.* 1995;61(suppl):621S–624S.

18. Fosmire GJ. Zinc toxicity. *Am J Clin Nutr.* 1990;51:225–227.

19. Dreno B, et al. Low doses of zinc gluconate for inflammatory acne. *Acta Derm Venereol.* 1989;69:541–543.

20. Pohit J, et al. Zinc status of acne vulgaris patients. *J Appl Nutr.* 1985;37:18–25.

21. Amer M, et al. Serum zinc in acne vulgaris. *Int J Dermatol.* 1982;21:481.

22. Michaëlsson G, et al. Serum zinc and retinol-binding protein in acne. *Br J Dermatol.* 1977;96:283–286.

23. Lidën S, et al. Clinical evaluation of acne. *Acta Derm Venereol.* 1980;89:49–52.

24. Michaëlsson G, Johlin L, Ljunghall K. A double-blind study of the effect of zinc and oxytetracycline in acne vulgaris. *Br J Dermatol.* 1997;97:561–566.

25. Dreno B, et al. 1989.

26. Verma KC, et al. Oral zinc sulfate therapy in acne vulgaris: a double blind trial. *Acta Dermatovener.* 1980;60:337.

27. Weimar VM, et al. Zinc sulfate in acne vulgaris. *Arch Dermatol.* 1978;114(12):1776–1778.

28. Göransson K, et al. Oral zinc in acne vulgaris: A clinical and methodological study. *Acta Derm Venereol.* 1978;58(5):443–448.

29. Hillström L, et al. Comparison of oral treatment with zinc sulphate and placebo in acne vulgaris. *Br J Dermatol.* 1977;97(6):679–684.

30. Gupta VL, Chaubey BS. Efficacy of zinc therapy in prevention of crisis in sickle-cell anemia: a double-blind, randomized controlled clinical trial. *J Assoc Physicians India.* 1995;43:467–469.

31. Simkin PA. Treatment of rheumatoid arthritis with oral zinc sulfate. *Agents Actions.* 1981;8:587–595.

32. Pandley SP, Bhattacharya SK, Sundar S. Zinc in rheumatoid arthritis. *Indian J Med Res.* 1985;81:618–620.

33. Mattingly PC, et al. Zinc sulphate in rheumatoid arthritis. *Ann Rheum Dis.* 1982;41:456–457.

34. Rasker JJ, Kardaun SH. Lack of beneficial effect of zinc sulphate in rheumatoid arthritis. *Scand J Rheumatol.* 1982;11:168–170.

35. Dixon JS, et al. Biochemical and clinical changes occurring during the treatment of rheumatoid arthritis with novel antirheumatoid drugs. *Int J Clin Pharmacol Res.* 1985;5(1):25–33.

36. Job C, et al. Zinc sulphate in the treatment of rheumatoid arthritis. *Arthritis Rheum.* 1980;23:1408.

37. Simkin PA. 1981.

38. Netter A, et al. Effect of zinc administration on plasma testosterone, dihydrotestosterone and sperm count. *Arch Androl.* 1981;7:69–73.

39. Stur M, et al. Oral zinc and the second eye in age-related macular degeneration. *Invest Ophthalmol Vis Sci.* 1993;37:1225–1235.

40. Newsome DA, et al. Oral zinc in macular degeneration. *Arch Ophthalmol.* 1988;106(2):192–198.

41. Frommer DJ. The healing of gastric ulcers by zinc sulphate. *Med J Aust.* 1975;2:793–796.

42. Garcia-Plaza A, et al. A multicenter clinical trial. Zinc acexamate versus famotidine in the treatment of acute duodenal ulcer [in Spanish]. *Rev Esp Enferm Dig.* 1996;88:757–762.

43. Bandlish U, Prabhakar BR, Wadehra PL. Plasma zinc level estimation in enlarged prostate. *Indian J Pathol Microbiol.* 1988;31(3):231–234.

44. Gonick P, et al. Atomic absorption spectrophotometric determination of zinc in the prostate. *Invest Urol.* 1969;6:345–347.

45. Schrodt GR, et al. The concentration of zinc in diseased human prostate glands. *Cancer.* 1964;17:1555–1566.

46. Györkey F, et al. Zinc and magnesium in human prostate gland: normal, hyperplastic and neoplastic. *Cancer Res.* 1967;27:1348–1353.

47. Györkey F, Sato CS. In vitro 65 zinc-binding capacities of normal hyperplastic and carcinomatous human prostate gland. *Exp Mol Pathol.* 1968;8:216–224.

48. Judd AM, et al. Zinc acutely, selectively and reversibly inhibits pituitary prolactin secretion. *Brain Res.* 1984;294:190–192.

49. Leake A, et al. Interaction between prolactin and zinc in the human prostate gland. *J Endocrinol.* 1984;102(1):73–76.

50. Leake A, Chisholm GD, Habib FK. The effect of zinc on the 5-alpha-reduction of testosterone by the hyperplastic human prostate gland. *J Steroid Biochem.* 1984;20:651–655.

51. Leake A, et al. Subcellular distribution of zinc in the benign and malignant human prostate: evidence for a direct zinc androgen interaction. *Acta Endocrinol (Copenh).* 1984;105:281–288.

52. Neal DE, et al. Changes in seminal fluid zinc during experimental prostatitis. *Urol Res.* 1993;21:71–74.

53. Rodger RS, et al. Zinc deficiency and hyperprolactinaemia are not reversible causes of sexual dysfunction in uraemia. *Nephrol Dial Transplant.* 1989;4:888–892.

54. Feustel A, Wennrich R. Zinc and cadmium plasma and erythro-cyte levels in prostatic carcinoma, BPH, urological malignancies, and inflammations. *Prostate.* 1986;8:75–79.

55. Goldenberg RL, et al. The effect of zinc supplementation on pregnancy outcome. *JAMA.* 1995;274:463–468.

56. Sustrova M, et al. Thyroid function and plasma immunoglobulins in subjects with Down's syndrome (DS) during ontogenesis and zinc therapy. *J Endocrinol Invest.* 1994;17:385–390.

57. Licastro F, et al. Modulation of the neuroendocrine system and immune functions by zinc supplementation in children with Down's syndrome. *J Trace Elem Electrolytes Health Dis.* 1993;7:237–239.

58. Lockitch G, et al. Infection and immunity in Down syndrome: a trial of long-term low oral doses of zinc. *J Pediatr.* 1989;114:781–787.

59. Constantinidis J. Alzheimer's disease and the zinc theory [in French]. *Encephale.* 1990;16:231–239.

60. Constantinidis J. The hypothesis of zinc deficiency in the patho-genesis of neurofibrillary tangles. *Med Hypotheses.* 1991;35:319–323.

61. Cuajungco MP, Lees GJ. Zinc metabolism in the brain: relevance to human neurodegenerative disorders. *Neurobiol Dis.* 1997;4:137–169.

62. Lovell MA, et al. Copper, iron and zinc in Alzheimer's disease senile plaques. *J Neurol Sci.* 1998;158:47–52.

63. Han CM. Changes in body zinc and copper levels in severely burned patients and the effects of oral administration of $ZnSO_4$ by a double-blind method. *Chung Hua Cheng Hsing Shao Shang Wai Ko Tsa Chih.* 1990;6:83–86,155.

64. Agren MS, et al. Selenium, zinc, iron and copper levels in serum of patients with arterial and venous leg ulcers. *Acta Derm Venereol.* 1986;66:237–240.

65. Floersheim GL, Lais E. Lack of effect of oral zinc sulfate on wound healing in leg ulcer [in German]. *Schweiz Med Wochen-schr.* 1980;110:1138–1145.

66. Sjögren A, Floren CH, Nilsson A. Evaluation of zinc status in subjects with Crohn's disease. *J Am Coll Nutr.* 1988;7:57–60.

67. Van de Wal Y, et al. Effect of zinc therapy on natural killer cell activity in inflammatory bowel disease. *Aliment Pharmacol Ther.* 1993;7:281–286.

68. Mulder TP, et al. Effect of oral zinc supplementation on metallothionein and superoxide dismutase concentrations in patients with inflammatory bowel disease. *J Gastroenterol Hepatol.* 1994;9:472–477.

69. Dronfield MW, Malone JD, Langman MJ. Zinc in ulcerative colitis: a therapeutic trial and report on plasma levels. *Gut.* 1977;18:33–36.

70. Gersdorff M, et al. The zinc sulfate overload test in patients suffering from tinnitus associated with low serum zinc. Preliminary report [in French]. *Acta Otorhinolaryngol Belg.* 1987;41:498–505.

71. Paaske PB, et al. Zinc therapy of tinnitus. A placebo-controlled study [in Danish]. *Ugeskr Laeger.* 1990;152:2473–2475.

72. Relea P, et al. Zinc, biochemical markers of nutrition, and type-I osteoporosis. *Age Ageing.* 1995;24:303–307.

73. Schmidt LE, Arfken CL, Heins JM. Evaluation of nutrient intake in subjects with non-insulin-dependent diabetes mellitus. *J Am Diet Assoc.* 1994;94:773–774.

74. Blostein-Fujii A, et al. Short-term zinc supplementation in women with non-insulin-dependent diabetes mellitus: effects on plasma 5'-nucleotidase activities, insulin-like growth factor I concentrations, and lipoprotein oxidation rates in vitro. *Am J Clin Nutr.* 1997;66:639–642.

75. Rauscher AM, et al. Zinc metabolism in non-insulin-dependent diabetes mellitus. *J Trace Elem Med Biol.* 1997;11:65–70.

76. Mocchegiani E, et al. Benefit of oral zinc supplementation as an adjunct to zidovudine (AZT) therapy against opportunistic infections in AIDS. *Int J Immunopharmacol.* 1995;17:719–727.

77. Birmingham CL, Goldner EM, Bakan R. Controlled trial of zinc supplementation in anorexia nervosa. *Int J Eat Disord.* 1994;15:251–255.

78. Katz RL, et al. Zinc deficiency in anorexia nervosa. *J Adolesc Health Care.* 1987;8:400–406.

79. Lask B, et al. Zinc deficiency and childhood-onset anorexia nervosa. *J Clin Psychiatry.* 1993;54:63–66.

80. Roijen SB, Worsaae U, Zlotnik G. Zinc in patients with anorexia nervosa [in Danish]. *Ugeskr Laeger.* 1991;153:721–723.

Andrographis: Eastern Medicine Moves West

1. Yarnell, E. Four major Ayurvedic herbs: a Western perspective. *Altern Complement Therap.* Oct. 1998;321–325.

2. Yarnell, E. 1998.

3. Hancke J, et al. A double-blind study with a new monodrug Kan Jang: Decrease of symptoms and improvements in the recovery from common colds. *Phytother Res.* 1995;9:559–562.

4. Melchior J, et al. Controlled clinical study of standardized *Andrographis paniculata* extract in common cold: a pilot trial. *Phytomedicine.* 1996–1997;34:314–318.

5. Hancke J, et al. 1995.

6. Thamlikitkul V, et al. Efficacy of *Andrographis paniculata* (Nees) for pharyngotonsillitis in adults. *J Med Assoc Thai.* 1991;74(10):437–442.

7. Puri A, et al. Immunostimulant agents from *Andrographis paniculata. J Nat Prod.* July 1993;56(7):995–9.

8. Zhang CY, Tan BK. Mechanisms of cardiovascular activity of *Andrographis paniculata* in the anaesthetized rat. *J Ethnopharmacol.* April 1997;56(2):97–101.

9. Choudhury BR, Poddar MK. Andrographolide and kalmegh (*Andrographis paniculata)* extract: in vivo and in vitro effect on hepatic lipid peroxidation. *Exp Clin Pharmacol.* September 1984;6(9):481–5;

10. Hancke J, et al. A double-blind study with a new monodrug Kan Jang: Decrease of symptoms and improvements in the recovery from common colds. *Phytother Res.* 1995;9:559–562.

11. Akbarsha MA, et al. Antifertility effect of *Andrographis panicu-lata* (Nees) in male albino rat. *Indian J Exp Biol.* 1990;28(5):421–426.

12. Burgos RA, et al. Testicular toxicity assessment of *Andrographis paniculata* dried extract in rats. *J Ethnopharmacol.* 1997;58(3):219–224.

13. Zoha MS, et al. Antifertility effect of *Andrographis paniculata* in mice. *Bangladesh Med Res Counc Bull.* 1989;15(1):34–37.

14. Choudhury BR, Poddar MK. Andrographolide and kalmegh *(Andrographis paniculata)* extract: in vivo and in vitro effect on hepatic lipid peroxidation. *Exp Clin Pharmacol.* September 1984;6(9):481–5.

15. Choudhury BR, Poddar MK. Effect of Kalmegh extract on rat liver and serum enzymes. *Methods Find Exp Clin Pharmacol.* December 1983;5(10):727–30.

16. Kapil A, et al. Antihepatotoxic effects of major diterpenoid con-stituents *of Andrographis paniculata. Biochem Pharmacol.* July 6, 1993;46(1):182–185.

17. Shukla B, et al. Choleretic effect of andrographolide in rats and guinea pigs. *Planta Med.* April 1992;58(2):146–149.

18. Rana AC, Avadhoot Y. Hepatoprotective effects of *Andrographis paniculata* against carbon tetrachloride–induced liver damage. *Arch Pharm Res.* March 1991;14(1):93–95.

19. Handa SS, Sharma A. Hepatoprotective activity of andro-grapholide from *Andrographis paniculata* against carbon-tetrachloride. *Indian J Med Res.* August 1990;92:276–83.

20. Handa SS, Sharma A. Hepatoprotective activity of andro-grapholide against galactosamine and paracetamol intoxication in rats. *Indian J Med Res.* August 1990;92:284–292.

21. Visen PK, et al. Andrographolide protects rat hepatocytes against paracetamol-induced damage. *J Ethnopharmacol.* October 1993;40(2):131–136.

22. Zhang CY, Tan BK. Mechanisms of cardiovascular activity of *An-drographis paniculata* in the anaesthetized rat. *J Ethnopharma-col.* 1997;56(2):97–101.

23. Zhang CY, Tan BK. Hypotensive activity of aqueous extract of *Andrographis paniculata* in rats. *Clin Exp Pharmacol Physiol.* 1996 August;23(8):675–678.

24. Zhang C, Kuroyangi M, Tan BK. Cardiovascular activity of 14-deoxy-11,12-didehydroandrographolide in the anaesthetised rat and isolated right atria. *Pharmacol Res.* December 1998;38(6):413–417.

25. Wang DW, Zhao HY. Experimental studies on prevention of atherosclerotic arterial stenosis and restenosis after angioplasty with *Andrographis Paniculata* Nees and fish oil. *J Tongji Med Univ.* 1993;13(4):193–198.

26. Wang DW, Zhao HY. Prevention of atherosclerotic arterial stenosis and restenosis after angioplasty with *Andrographis paniculata* nees and fish oil. Experimental studies of effects and mechanisms. *Chin Med J* (English). June 1994;107(6):464–70.

27. Guo ZL, Zhao HY, Zheng XH. The effect of *Andrographis paniculata* nees (APN) in alleviating the myocardial ischemic reperfusion injury. *J Tongji Med Univ.* 1994;14(1):49–51.

28. Guo Z, Zhao H, Fu L. Protective effects of API0134 on myocardial ischemia and reperfusion injury. *J Tongji Med Univ.* 1996;16(4):193–7.

29. Guo ZL, Zhao HY, Zheng XH. An experimental study of the mechanism of *Andrographis paniculata* nees (APN) in alleviating the Ca(2+)-overloading in the process of myocardial ischemic reperfusion. *J Tongji Med Univ.* 1995;15(4):205–8.

30. Zhao HY, Fang WY. Protective effects of *Andrographis paniculata* nees on post-infarction myocardium in experimental dogs. *J Tongji Med Univ.* 1990;10(4):212–7.

31. Zhao HY, Fang WY. Antithrombotic effects of *Andrographis paniculata* Nees in preventing myocardial infarction. *Chin Med J* (English). September 1991;104(9):770–5.

32. Najib Nik A, et al. Antimalarial activity of extracts of Malaysian medicinal plants. *J Ethnopharmacol.* March 1999;64(3):249–54.

33. Raj RK. Screening of indigenous plants for anthelmintic action against human *Ascaris lumbricoides:* Part II. *Indian J Physiol Pharmacol.* January–March 1975;19(1).

34. Dutta A, Sukul NC. Filaricidal properties of a wild herb, *Andrographis paniculata. J Helminthol.* June 1982;56(2):81–4.

35. Leelarasamee A, Trakulsomboon S, Sittisomwong N. Undetectable anti-bacterial activity of *Andrographis paniculata* (Burma) wall. *J Med Assoc Thai.* June 1990;73(6):299–304.

36. Gozalbes R, et al. Molecular search of new active drugs against *Toxoplasma gondii. SAR QSAR Environ Res.* 1999;10(1):47–60.

Other Herbs and Supplements for Colds: An Alternative Potpourri

1. Zakay-Rones Z, et al. Inhibition of several strains of influenza virus and reduction of symptoms by an elderberry extract (*Sambucus nigra* L.) during an outbreak of influenza B Panama. *J Altern Complement Med.* 1995;1(4):361–369.

2. Shapira-Nahor B, et al. The effect of Sambucol on HIV infection in vitro. Annual Israel Congress of Microbiology. February 6–7, 1995.

3. Morag A, et al. Inhibition of sensitive and acyclovir-resistant HSV-1 strains by an elderberry extract in vitro. *Xth International Congress of Virology.* Jerusalem; 1996: abstract 18–23.

4. Bensky D, Gamble A. *Chinese herbal medicine: Materia medica.* Seattle, WA: Eastland Press; 1986:383–384.

5. Moore M. *Medicinal plants of the mountain west.* Santa Fe, NM: Museum of New Mexico Press; 1979:119.

6. Tyler V. *The honest herbal.* 3rd ed. Binghamton, New York: Pharmaceutical Products Press; 1993:219–220.

7. Somerville KW, et al. Stones in the common bile duct: experience with medical dissolution therapy. *Postgrad Med J.* 1985;61:313–316.

8. *Review of Natural Products.* Yerba santa *monograph.* St. Louis, MO: Facts and Comparisons, Division, J.B. Lippincott Company; 1991.

9. *Review of Natural Products.* 1991.

10. Tierra M. *The way of herbs.* New York: Pocket Books; 1990:254.

11. Newall C, et al. *Herbal medicines: A guide for health-care professionals.* London: Pharmaceutical Press; 1996:188.

12. Tomodo M, et al. Hypoglycemic activity of twenty plant mucilages and three modified products. *Planta Med.* 1987;53:8–12.

13. Newall C, et al. 1996.

14. Sumiyoshi H. New pharmacological activities of garlic and its constituents [in Japanese]. *Nippon Yakurigaku Zasshi.* 1997;110(suppl 1):93P–97P.

Adaptogens for Colds and Flus: Potential for Prevention

1. Scaglione F, et al. Efficacy and safety of the standardised ginseng extract G115 for potentiating vaccination against the influenza syndrome and protection against the common cold. *Drugs Exp Clin Res.* 1996;22(2):65–72.

2. Brekhman II. *Eleutheroccoccus*: 20 years of research and clinical application. 1st International symposium on *Eleutherococcus.* Hamburg, Germany; 1980. Cited by: Brown D. *Herbal prescriptions for better health.* Rocklin, CA: Prima Publishing; 1997.

3. Schulz V, et al. *Rational phytotherapy.* 3rd ed. New York: Springer-Verlag; 1998:273.

4. Scaglione F, et al. 1996.

5. Awang, DVC. Maternal use of ginseng and neonatal androgenization. *JAMA.* 1991;266:363.

6. Ploss E. *Panax ginseng.* In C.A. Meyer. *Scientific report.* Cologne: Kooperation Phytopharmaka; 1988.

7. *Lawrence Review of Natural Products. Ginseng monograph.* St. Louis: Facts and Comparisons Division, J.B. Lippincott Company; 1990.

8. Tyler V. *Herbs of choice.* New York: Haworth Press; 1994.

9. Scaglione F, et al. 1986.

10. Baldwin CA, et al. What pharmacists should know about ginseng. *Pharm J.* 1986;237:583–610.

11. Tyler V. 1994.

12. Siegel RK. Ginseng abuse syndrome. Problems with the panacea. *JAMA.* 1979;241:1614–1615.

13. Tyler V. 1994.

14. Schulz V, et al. 1998.

15. Kroll D. University of Colorado School of Pharmacy. Unpublished communication. 1998.

16. Jones BD, et al. Interaction of ginseng with phenelzine. *J Clin Psychopharmacol.* 1987;7:201–202.

17. Janetzky K, Morreale AP. Probable interaction between warfarin and ginseng. *Am J Health Syst Pharm.* 1997;54:692–693.

18. McRae S. Elevated serum digoxin levels in a patient taking digoxin and Siberian ginseng. *Can Med Assoc J.* 1996;155(3):293–295.

19. Sotaneimi EA, et al. Ginseng therapy in non-insulin–dependent diabetic patients. *Diabetes Care.* 1995;18(10):1373–1375.

20. Sorenson H, et al. A double-masked study of the effects of ginseng on cognitive functions. *Curr Ther Res Clin Exp.* 1996;57(12):959–968.

21. Dowling EA, et al. Effect of *Eleutherococcus senticosus* on submaximal and maximal exercise performance. *Med Sci Sports Exerc.* 1996;28(4):482–489.

22. Enles HJ, Wirth JC. No ergogenic effects of ginseng (*Panax ginseng*, C. A. Meyer) during graded maximal aerobic exercise. *J Am Diet Assoc.* 1997;97:1110–1115.

23. Yun TK, Choi SY. Non-organ specific cancer prevention of ginseng: A prospective study in Korea. *Int J Epidemiol.* 1998;27:359–364.

24. Bensky D, Gamble A. *Chinese herbal medicine: Materia medica.* Seattle, WA: Eastland Press; 1986:457–459.

25. Hou Y, et al. Effect of *Radix Astragali Seu Hedysari* on the interferon system. *Chin Med J.* 1981;94:35–40.

26. Sun Y, et al. Immune restoration and/or augmentation of local graft versus host reaction by traditional Chinese medicinal herbs. *Cancer.* 1983;52:70–73.

27. Bensky D, Gamble A. 1986.

28. Bensky D, Gamble A. 1986.

29. Liang R, et al. Clinical study on braincalming tablets in treating 450 cases of atherosclerosis. *J North Chin Med.* 1985;1:63–65.

30. Xiao S, et al. Hyperthyroidism treated with yiqiyangyin decoction. *J Trad Chin Med.* 1986;6(2):79–82.

31. Zhang ND, et al. Effects on blood pressure and inflammation of astragalus saponin 1, a principle isolated from *Astragalus membranaceus* Bge. *Acta Pharm Suec.* 1984;19(5):333–337.

32. Zhang H, et al. Treatment of adult diabetes with jiangtangjia tablets. *J Trad Chin Med.* 1986;7(4):37–39.

33. Zhou MX, et al. Therapeutic effect of astragalus in treating chronic active hepatitis and the changes in immune function. *J Chin People's Liberation Army.* 1982;7(4):242–244.

34. Dhuley JN. Therapeutic efficacy of *Ashwagandha* against experimental aspergillosis in mice. *Immunopharmacol Immunotoxicol.* 1998;20(1):191–198.

35. Lindner, S. *Withania somnifera. Aust J Med Herbalism.* 1996;8(3)78–82.

36. Devi PU, et al. In vivo growth inhibitory effect of *Withania somnifera* (ashwaganda) on a transplantable mouse tumour, Sarcoma 180. *Indian J Exp Biol.* 1992;30:169–172.

37. Al-Hindawi MK, et al. Anti-granuloma activity of Iraqi *Withania somnifera. J Ethnopharmacol.* 1992;37:113–116.

38. Kuppurajan K, et al. Effect of ashwaganda (*Withania somnifera* Dunal) on the process of aging in human volunteers. *J Res Ayurveda Siddha.* 1980;1:247–258.

39. Bone K. *MediHerb Professional Newsletter* No. 30, Warwick, Australia; 1998.

40. Yamada Y, et al. Antitumor effect of orally administered extracts from fruit body of *Grifola frondosa* (maitake). *Chemotherapy.* 1990;38:790–796.

41. Nanba H. Immunostimulant activity in vivo and anti-HIV activity in vitro of 3 branched b-1-6-glucans extracted from maitake mushrooms (*Grifola frondosa*). (abstract). Amsterdam: VIII International Conference on AIDS; 1992.

42. De Oliveira F. *Pfaffia paniculata* (Martius) Kuntze–Brazilian ginseng. *Rev Bras Farmacog.* 1986;1(1):86–92.

43. Melchart, D, et al. Echinacea root extracts for the prevention of upper respiratory tract infections: a double-blind, placebo-controlled randomized trial. *Arch Fam Med.* 1998;7:541–545.

44. Melchart D, et al. Immunomodulation with echinacea: a systematic review of controlled clinical trials. *Phytomedicine.* 1994;1:245–254. Cited by: Schulz V, et al. *Rational phytotherapy.* 3rd ed. New York: Springer-Verlag; 1998:276.

45. Schoneberger D. The influence of immune-stimulating effects of pressed juice from *Echinacea purpurea* on the course and severity of colds. *Forum Immunol.* 1992; 8:2–12. Translated by Sigrid M Klein. 1993.

46. Chamberlain, C. Popular herb may make colds worse. http://www.abcnews.go.com/sections/living/Daily News/echinacea990427.html

Vitamins, Minerals, and Andrographis for Prevention

1. Cáceres J, et al. Prevention of common colds with *Andrographis paniculata* dried extract: a pilot double blind trial. *Phytomedicine.* 1997;4(2):101–104.

2. Christen S, et al. Gamma-tocopherol traps mutagenic electrophiles such as NOX and complements alpha-tocopherol: physiological implications. *Proc Natl Acad Sci USA.* 1997;94:3217–3222.

3. Kiyose C, et al. Biodiscrimination of alpha-tocopherol stereoisomers in humans after oral administration. *Am J Clin Nutr.* March 1997;65(3):785–789.

4. Burton GW, et al. Human plasma and tissue alpha-tocopherol concentrations in response to supplementation with deuterated

natural and synthetic vitamin E. *Am J Clin Nutr.* April 1998;67(4):669–684.

5. Meydani SM, et al. Vitamin E supplementation and in vivo immune response in healthy elderly subjects: A randomized controlled trial. *JAMA.* 1997;277:1380–1386.

6. *Harrison's principles of internal medicine.* 14th ed. New York: McGraw-Hill; 1998.

7. Sanstead H. Zinc nutrition in the United States. *Am J Clin Nutr.* 1973;B26:1251–1260.

8. Prasad AS. Role of zinc in human health. *Contemp Nutr.* 1991:16(5):558–60.

9. Baum MK, et al. Zidovudine-associated adverse reactions in a longitudinal study of asymptomatic HIV-1 infected homosexual males. *J Acquir Immune Defic Syndr.* 1991;4(12):1218–1226.

10. Wardlaw GM. *Perspectives in nutrition.* St. Louis: Mosby; 1993:469.

11. Girodon F, et al. Effect of micronutrient supplementation on infection in institutionalized elderly subjects: a controlled trial. *Ann Nutr Metab.* 1997;41(2):98–107.

12. Sugarman B. Zinc and infection. *Rev Infect Dis.* 1983;5(1):137–147.

13. Sazawal S, et al. Zinc supplementation. *Pediatrics.* 1998;102(1).

14. Navert B, et al. A reduction of the phytate content of bran by leavening in bread and its effect on zinc absorption in man. *Br J Nutr.* 1985;53:47–53.

15. Vohra P, et al. Phytic acid-metal complexes. *Proc Soc Exp Biol Med.* 1965;120:447–449.

16. Hoffman HN II, et al. Zinc-induced copper deficiency. *Gastroenterology.* 1988;94:508–512.

17. Sandstead HH. Requirements and toxicity of essential trace elements, illustrated by zinc and copper. *Am J Clin Nutr.* 1995;61(suppl.):621S–624S.

18. Sanstead H. 1973.

19. Prasad AS. Role of zinc in human health. *Contemp Nutr.* 1991:16(5).

20. Hemilä H. Vitamin C intake and susceptibility to the common cold. *BMJ.* 1997;77(1):59–72.

21. Peters EM, et al. Vitamin C supplementation reduces the incidence of postrace symptoms of upper-respiratory-tract infection in ultramarathon runners. *Am J Clin Nutr.* 1993;57(2):170–174.

22. Hemilä H. Does vitamin C alleviate symptoms of the common cold? A review of current evidence. *Scand J Infect Dis.* 1994;26:1–6.

23. Hemilä H. Vitamin C and common cold incidence: a review of studies with subjects under heavy physical stress. *Int J Sports Med.* 1996;17(5):379–383.

24. Hemilä H. 1996.

25. Auer BL, et al. Relative hyperoxaluria, crystalluria, and hematuria after mega-dose ingestion of vitamin C. *Eur J Clin Invest.* 1998;28:695–700.

Lifestyle Changes for Prevention

1. Bartok L. Bacterial endotoxins and nonspecific resistance. *Acta Microbiol Immunol Hung.* 1997;44(4):361–5.

2. Sali A. Psychoneuroimmunology: fact or fiction? *Aust Fam Physician.* November 26, 1997;(11):1291–4, 1296–1299.

3. *Harrison's principles of internal medicine.* 14th ed. New York: McGraw-Hill; 1998.

4. Chandra RK. Nutrition and immunity: lessons from the past and new insights into the future. *Am J Clin Nutr.* 1991;53(5):1087–1101.

5. Anderson R, Theron A. Effects of B-complex vitamins on cellular and humoral immune functions in vitro and in vivo. *Int J Vitam Nutr Res.* 1983;24:77–84. Cited by: Werbach M. *Nutritional influences on illness.* 2nd ed. Tarzana, CA: Third Line Press; 1993.

6. Levy JA. Nutrition and the immune system, in Stiles DP, et al. *Basic and Clinical Immunology.* 4th ed. Los Altos, CA: Lange

Medical Publications; 1982:297–305. Cited by: Werbach M. *Nutritional Influences on Illness.* 2nd ed. Tarzana, CA: Third Line Press; 1993.

7. Beisel WR. Single nutrients and immunity. *Am J Clin Nutr.* 1982;35(suppl):417–468. Cited by: Werbach M. *Nutritional Influences on Illness.* 2nd ed. Tarzana, CA: Third Line Press; 1993.

8. Beisel WR, et al. Single-nutrient effects on immunologic functions. *JAMA.* 1981;245(1):53–58. Cited by: Werbach M. *Nutritional influences on illness.* 2nd ed. Tarzana, CA: Third Line Press; 1993.

9. Levy JA. 1982.

10. Chandra RK. 1991.

11. Chandra RK. 1991.

12. Pocino M, et al. Influence of oral administration of excess copper on the immune response. *Fundam Appl Toxicol.* 1991;16:249–256. Cited by: Werbach M. *Nutritional influences on illness.* 2nd ed. Tarzana, CA: Third Line Press; 1993.

13. Cohen S, et al. Smoking, alcohol consumption, and susceptibility to the common cold. *Am J Public Health.* September 1993;83(9): 1277–83.

14. Bernstein J, et al. Depression of lymphocyte transformation following oral glucose ingestion. *Am J Clin Nutr.* 1977;30:613. Cited by: Werbach M. *Nutritional influences on illness.* 2nd ed. Tarzana, CA: Third Line Press; 1993:354–355.

15. Nalder BN, et al. Sensitivity of the immunological response to the nutritional status of rats. *J Nutr.* 1972;102(4):535–541. Cited by: Werbach M. *Nutritional influences on illness.* 2nd ed. Tarzana, CA: Third Line Press; 1993:355.

16. Sanchez A, et al. Role of sugars in human neutrophilic phagocytosis. *Am J Clin Nutr.* 1973;26:180. Cited by: Werbach M. *Nutritional influences on illness.* 2nd ed. Tarzana, CA: Third Line Press; 1993:355.

17. Melamed I, et al. Coffee and the immune system. *Int J Immunol.* 1990;12:129–134. Cited by: Werbach M. *Nutritional influences on illness.* 2nd ed. Tarzana, CA: Third Line Press; 1993:355.

18. Kraal JH. Immunoglobulin levels in relation to smoking and coffee consumption. *Am J Clin Nutr* 1972; 31(2):198–200. Cited by: Werbach M. *Nutritional influences on illness.* 2nd ed. Tarzana, CA: Third Line Press; 1993:355.

Medications for Colds and Flus

1. *Harrison's principles of internal medicine.* 14th ed. New York: McGraw-Hill; 1998.

2. Stolberg SG. Federal agency approves anti-flu drug. *New York Times.* July 28, 1999: section A:14, col. 1.

3. Grady D. F.D.A. revising guidelines on antibiotics for animals. *The New York Times.* March 8, 1999.

4. Haney, DQ. New antibiotic hailed as able to take on resistant germs. (AP article in) *Fort Collins Coloradoan.* September 28, 1999.

Index

Visit Us at TNP.com

Andrographis *(continued)*
  for reducing duration of flus, 10
  for reducing symptoms of colds, 10, 52–53
  for reducing symptoms of flus, 10
  safety issues, 56–57
  studies, 52–53
Andrographolide in andrographis, 54
Anemia, zinc safety issue, 48
Anergy, 24
Anesthetic, local, peppermint as, 65
Animal feeds, antibiotics in, 118, 119
Anorexia
  immune deficiency from, 107
  zinc for, 49
Antibiotics
  andrographis as, 58
  in animal feeds, 118, 119
  bacteria resistant to, 118–119
  garlic as topical antibiotic, 70
  goldenseal as, 71
  ineffectiveness for colds and flus, 19–20, 119–120
  overuse of, 118–119
Antigens, 114
Antihistamines
  over-the-counter medicines, 118
  vitamin C as, 35
Anti-inflammatory drugs, vitamin C deficiency and, 36
Antioxidants
  cancer chemotherapy and, 40
  overview, 35
Antiviral drugs, 7, 116–117
Anxiety
  ashwagandha for, 85
  suma for, 88
Aphrodisiac, suma as, 88
Appetite enhancement, osha root for, 63
Arabinogalactan in echinacea, 27
Arabinoglactan in echinacea, 27
Ashwagandha, 12, 83–85
Asian ginseng. *See* Ginseng
Aspirin. *See also* Blood-thinning drugs
  garlic safety issue, 71

  for reducing symptoms of colds and flus, 117
  vitamin C deficiency and, 36
  vitamin E safety issue, 95
Asthma
  flu danger for, 3
  marshmallow for, 67
  reishi for, 87
  vitamin C for, 39
  yerba santa for, 66
Astragalus, 12, 81–83
Atherosclerosis prevention, andrographis for, 57
Atherosclerosis treatment, astragalus for, 83
Autoimmune diseases
  echinacea safety issue, 25, 29
  reishi for, 87
Ayurvedic medicine, andrographis in, 51
AZT, zinc absorption and, 97

B
Bacteria, 6, 118–119
Bacterial infections
  antibiotics and, 119
  flus and colds vs., 3
  secondary, 5–6, 7, 45–46
  viruses and susceptibility, 5–6, 7
  zinc for avoiding, 5–6, 10, 45–46
Bastyr College, 89
Bedsores, vitamin C for, 39
Ben-Gay, 65
Benign prostatic hyperplasia, zinc for, 49
Beta-D-glucan in maitake, 86
Bitters, king of. *See* Andrographis
Bladder infections
  vitamin C and, 39, 40
  zinc for, 49
Blinded placebo-controlled studies, 14–15
Bloating, as garlic side effect, 71
Blood-thinning drugs
  garlic safety issue, 71
  ginseng reaction with, 79
  reishi safety issue, 87

About the Authors

Anna M. Barton holds a degree in biological sciences. Her background includes work in biomedical research laboratories, freelance writing, and medical transcription. Her familiarity with these areas, combined with painstaking research, allows her to provide reliable information about alternatives and adjuncts to the standard western medical approach.

Elizabeth Collins, N.D., is a graduate of Reed College and the National College of Naturopathic Medicine. She practices family medicine and natural childbirth and also teaches at the National College of Naturopathic Medicine. Dr. Collins lives with her husband, David, in Portland, Oregon.

Nancy Berkoff, R.D., Ed.D., is a registered dietician, food technologist, and certified chef. She divides her time between teaching nutrition and culinary arts, food writing, and consulting.

About the Series Editors

Steven Bratman, M.D., is medical director for TNP.com. Dr. Bratman is both a strong proponent and vocal critic of alternative treatment, and he believes that alternative medicine has both strengths and weaknesses, just like conventional medicine. This even-handed critique has made him a trusted party on both sides of the debate. He has been an expert consultant to the State of Washington Medical Board, the Colorado Board of Medical Examiners, and the Texas State Board of Medical Examiners, evaluating disciplinary cases involving alternative medicine.

His books include *The Alternative Medicine Sourcebook: A Realistic Evaluation of Alternative Healing Methods* (1997), *The Alternative Medicine Ratings Guide: An Expert Panel Ranks the Best Alternative Treatments for Over 80 Conditions* (Prima Health, 1998), the professional text *Clinical Evaluation of Medicinal Herbs and Other Therapeutic Natural Products* (Prima Health, 1999), and the following titles in THE NATURAL PHARMACIST series: *Your Complete Guide to Herbs* (Prima Health, 1999), *Your Complete Guide to Illnesses and Their Natural Remedies* (Prima Health, 1999), *Natural Health Bible* (Prima Health, 1999), and *St. John's Wort and Depression* (Prima Health, 1999).

David J. Kroll, Ph.D., is a professor of pharmacology and toxicology at the University of Colorado School of Pharmacy and a consultant for pharmacists, physicians, and alternative practitioners on the indications and cautions for herbal medicine use. He received a degree in toxicology from the Philadelphia College of Pharmacy and Science and obtained his Ph.D. from the University of Florida College of Medicine. Dr. Kroll has lectured widely and has published articles in a number of medical journals, abstracts, and newsletters.

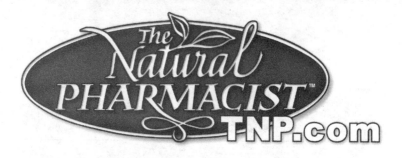

Science-Based Natural Health Information You Can Trust™

TNP.com Is:

- Science-based
- Independent and unbiased
- Up to date
- Balanced—offers both positive and negative findings
- Integrative—includes both conventional and natural treatments
- M.D. and Ph.D. supervised

From Asian Ginseng to Zinc, TNP.com cuts through the hype and tells you what is scientifically proven and what remains unknown about popular natural treatments. Setting a new, high standard of accuracy and objectivity, this Web site takes a realistic look at the herbs and supplements you hear about in the news and provides the balanced information necessary to make informed decisions about your health needs. If you want to be an informed consumer of natural products, TNP.com is the place to start.

Using TNP.com is easy, free, and private. Visit TNP.com now to get science-based natural health information you can trust!

Visit us online at www.TNP.com